Psychopathology - An International and Interdisciplinary Perspective

Edited by Robert Woolfolk, Lesley Allen, Federico Durbano and Floriana Irtelli

Published in London, United Kingdom

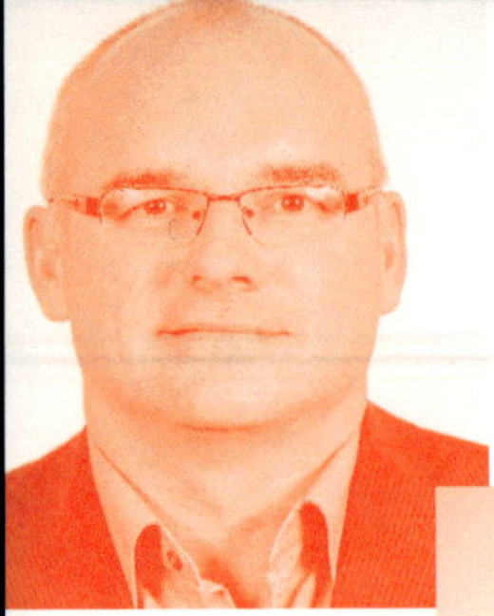
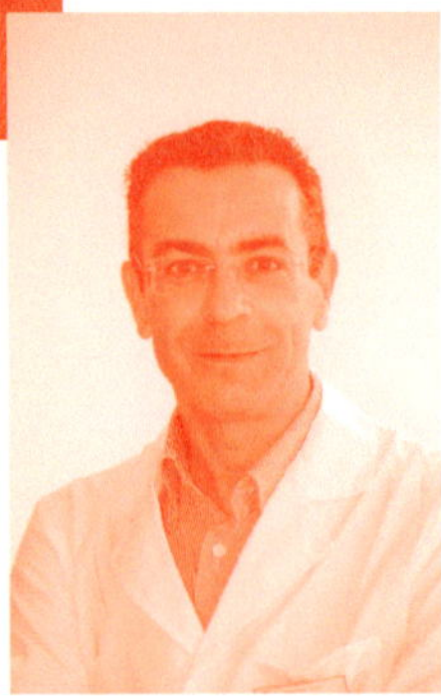
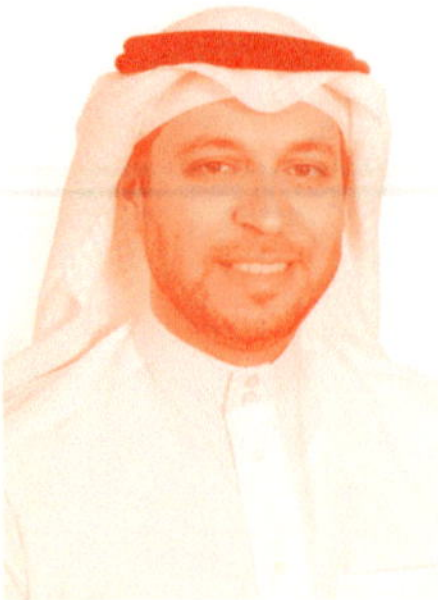
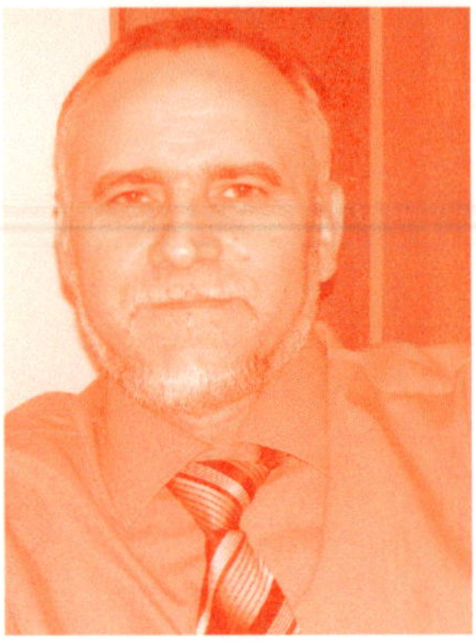
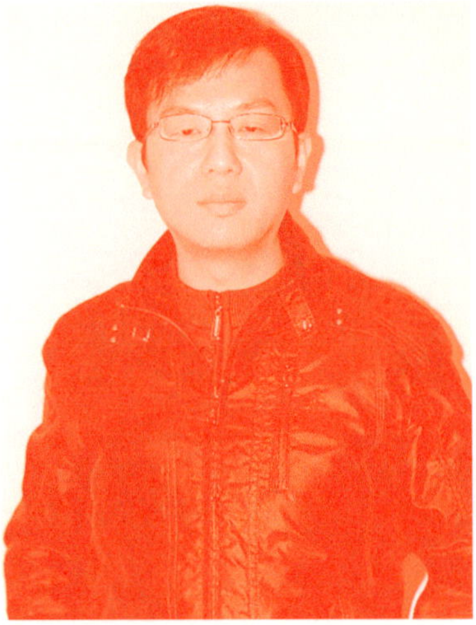
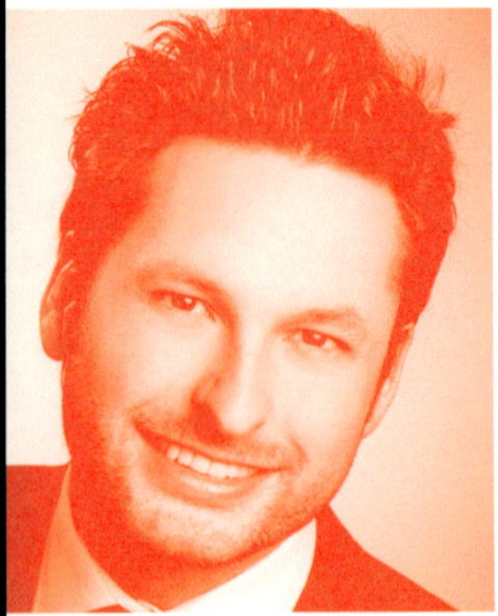
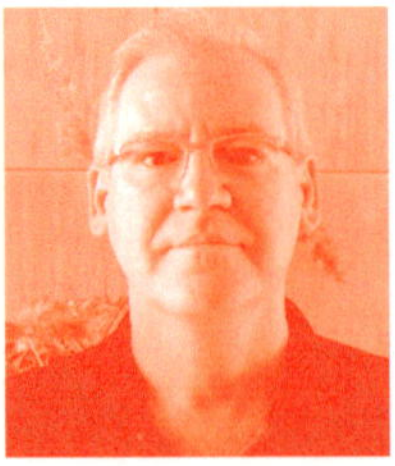

IntechOpen

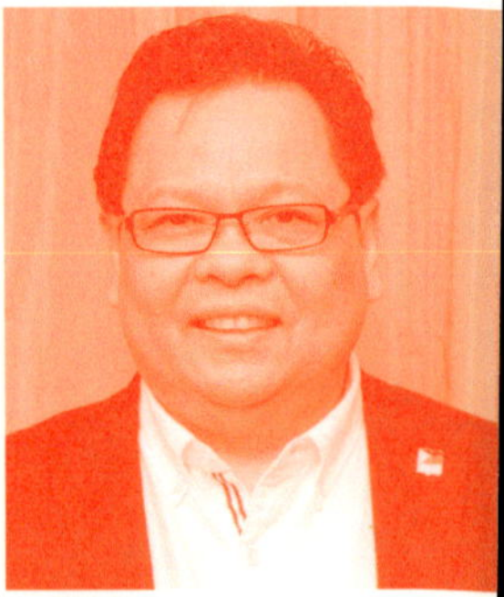
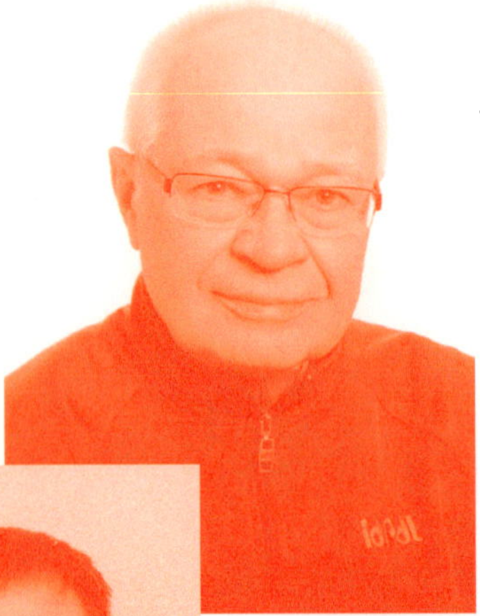
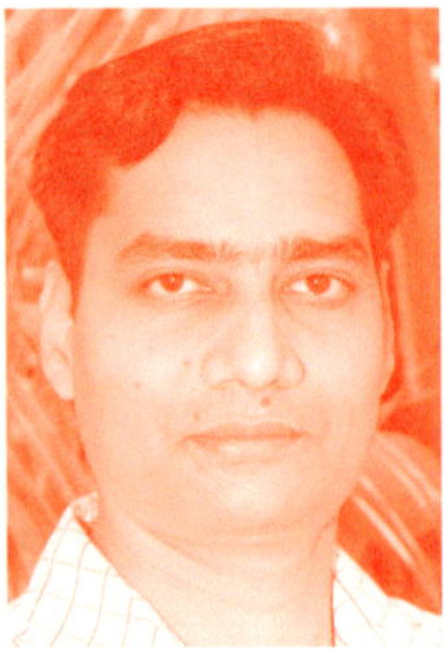
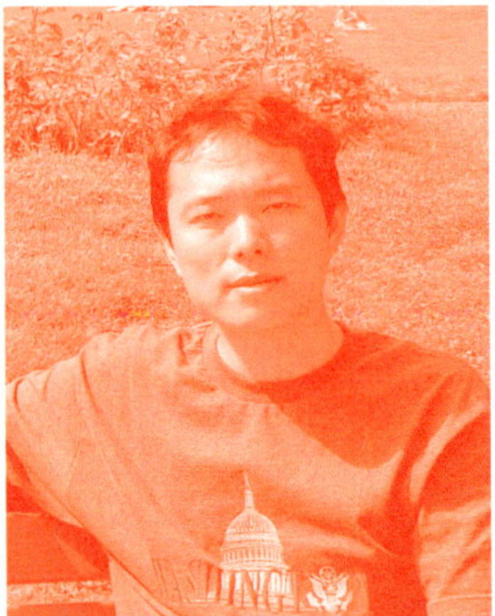
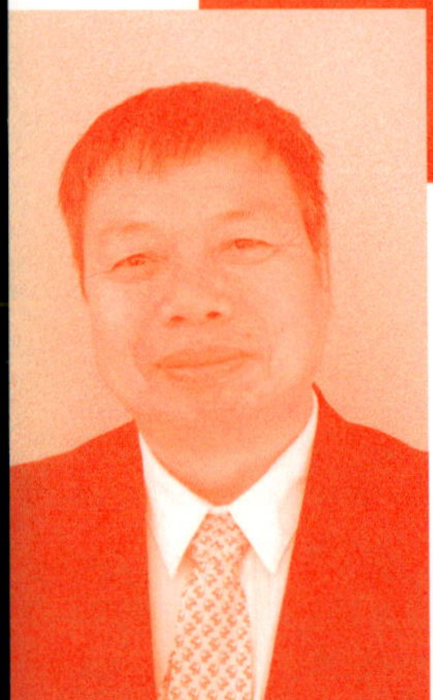
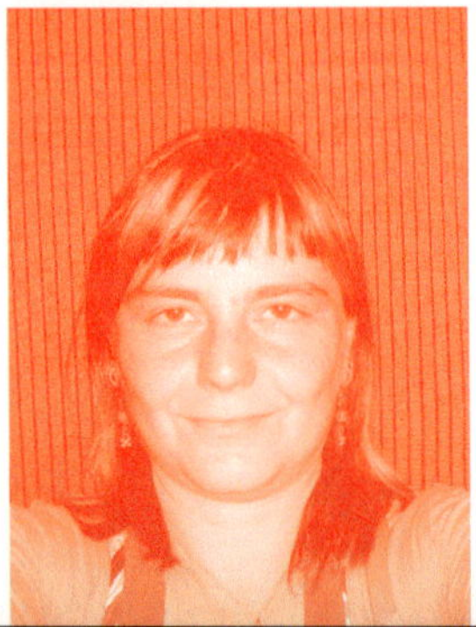

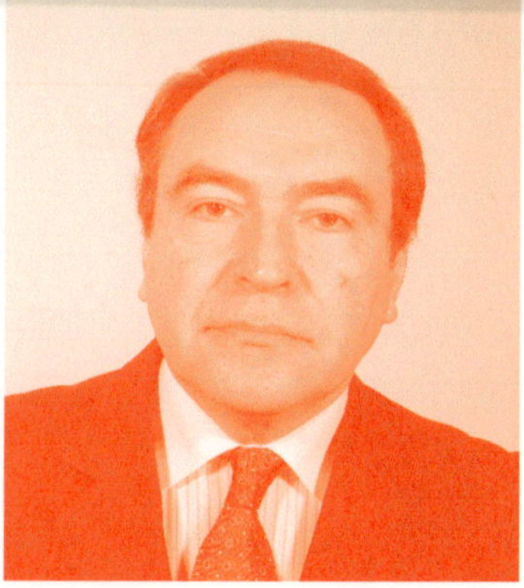
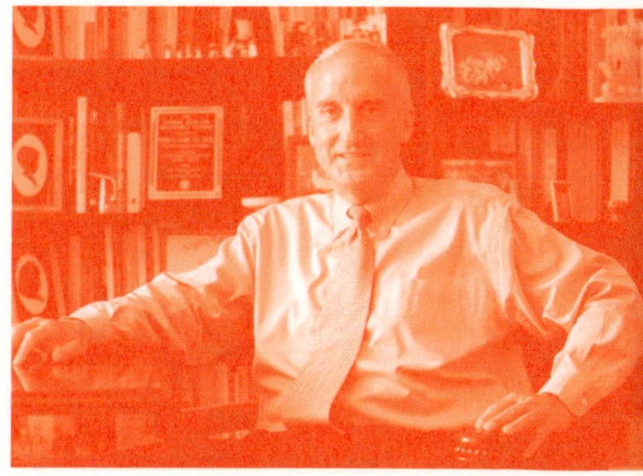
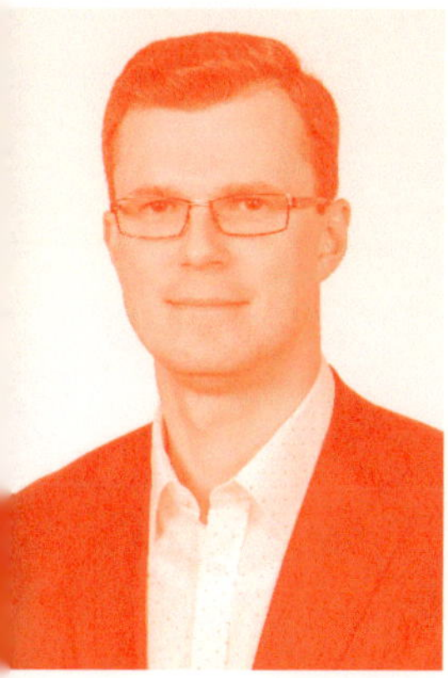
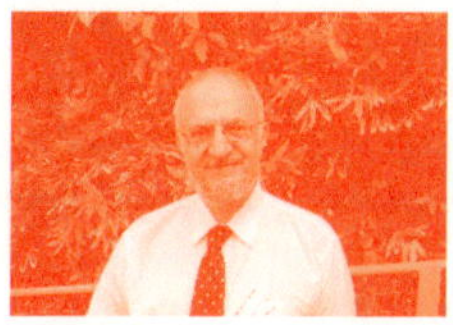
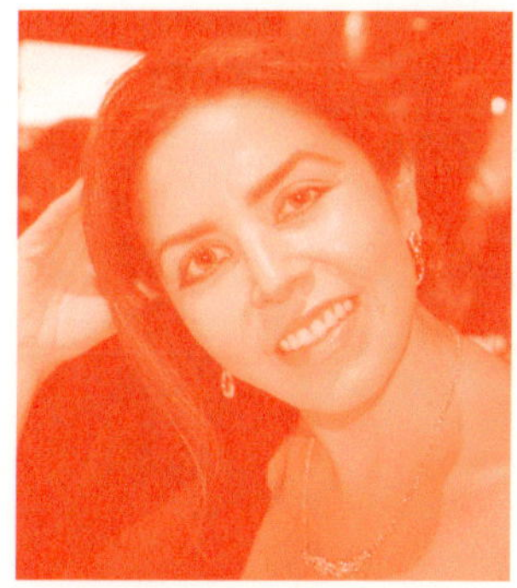

Supporting open minds since 2005

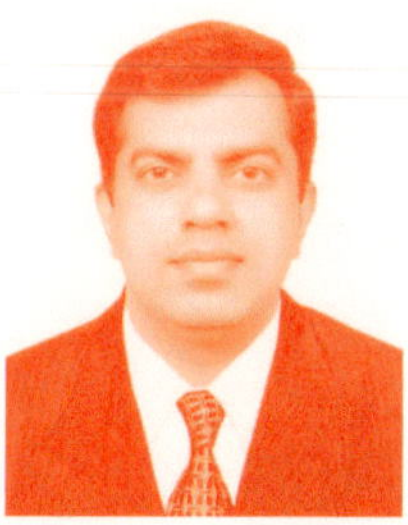
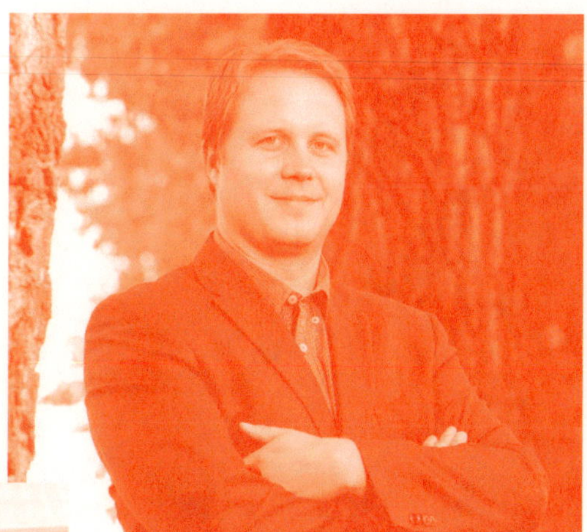
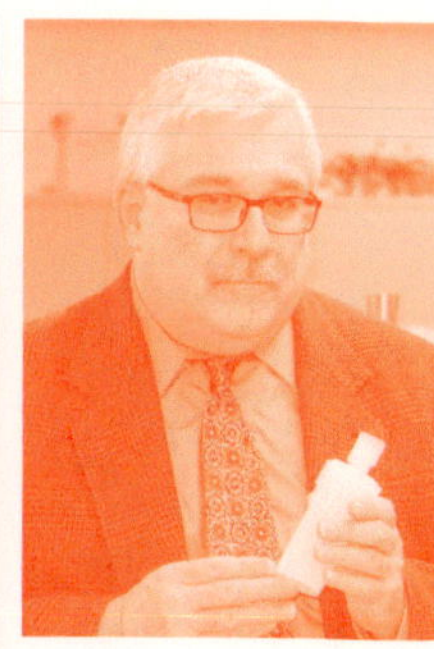
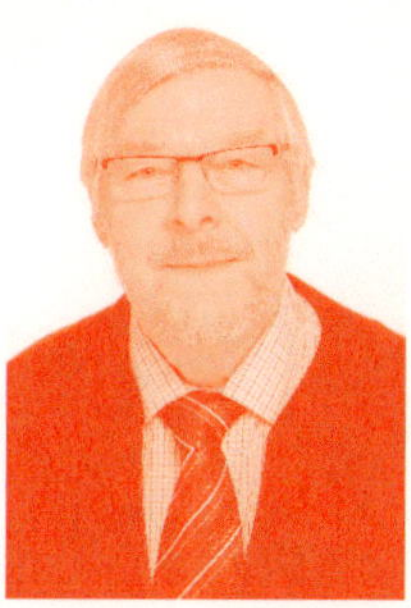
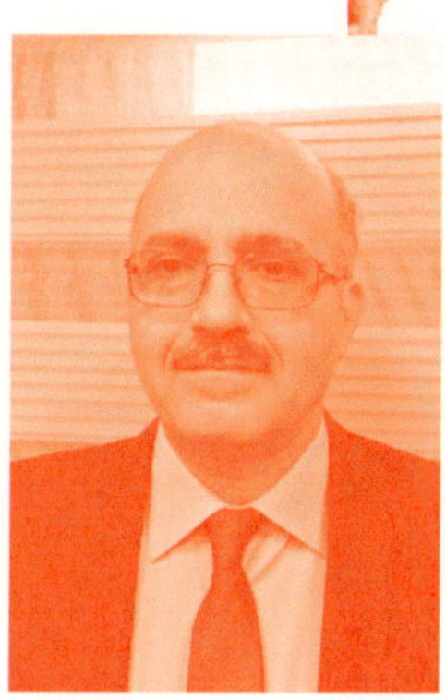
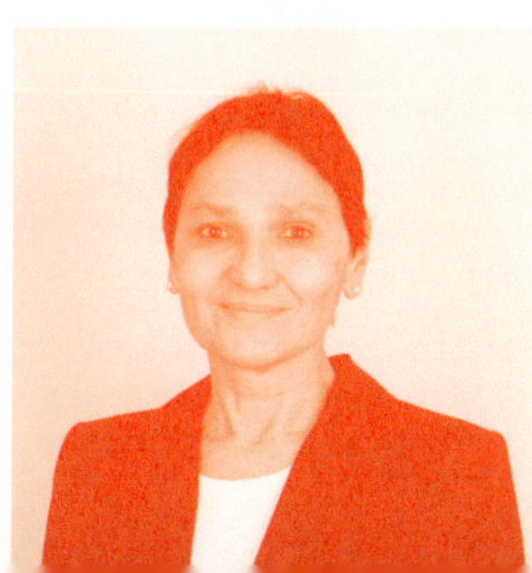
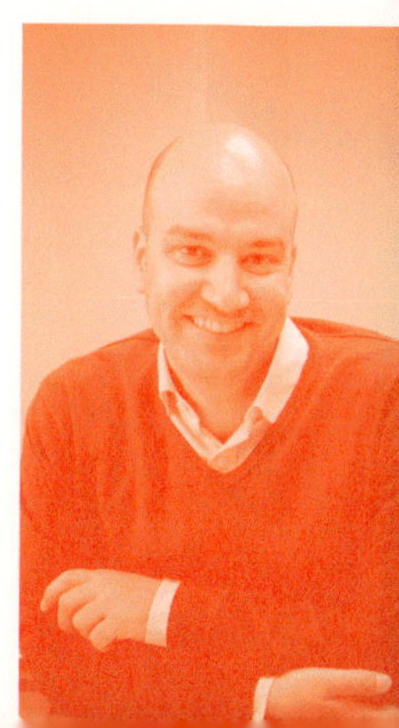

Psychopathology - An International and Interdisciplinary Perspective
http://dx.doi.org/10.5772/intechopen.73949
Edited by Robert Woolfolk, Lesley Allen, Federico Durbano and Floriana Irtelli

Contributors
Marie-Odile Soyer-Gobillard, charles sultan, Antonio Castro Neto, Magda Figueiroa, Renata Almeida, Rossana Rameh-De-Albuquerque, Iandê Moura, Solange Nappo, Martin Lorenzo Vargas, Ichitovkina Elena, Zlokazova Marina, Andrey Soloviev, Elena Predescu, Anna Boglarka Asztalos, Roxana Sipos, Robert Woolfolk, Geneviève Belleville, Alenka Potočnik, Dimitar Bonevski, Andromahi Naumovska, Peter Slater, Fernando Oliveira Costa, Fabiano Cunha, Rafael Lima

First published in London, United Kingdom, 2020 by IntechOpen
IntechOpen is the global imprint of INTECHOPEN LIMITED, registered in England and Wales, registration number: 11086078, 7th floor, 10 Lower Thames Street, London, EC3R 6AF, United Kingdom
Printed in Croatia

British Library Cataloguing-in-Publication Data
A catalogue record for this book is available from the British Library

Additional hard and PDF copies can be obtained from orders@intechopen.com

Psychopathology - An International and Interdisciplinary Perspective
Edited by Robert Woolfolk, Lesley Allen, Federico Durbano and Floriana Irtelli
p. cm.
Print ISBN 978-1-78985-819-8
Online ISBN 978-1-78985-820-4
eBook (PDF) ISBN 978-1-83880-019-2

For EU product safety concerns:
IN TECH d.o.o., Prolaz Marije Krucifikse Kozulić 3, 51000 Rijeka, Croatia, info@intechopen.com or visit our website at intechopen.com.

Meet the editors

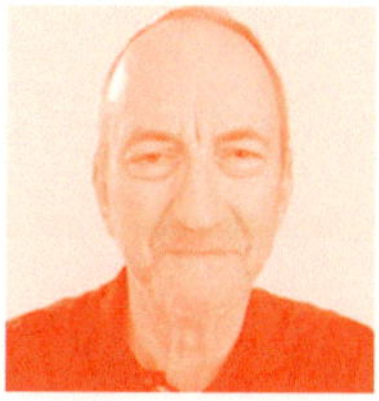

Robert L. Woolfolk, PhD, is Professor of Psychology and Philosophy at Rutgers University. He has served on the faculties of Princeton University and the University of Texas at Austin. He has published numerous papers and several books on psychotherapy, psychopathology, and the philosophical foundations of psychology. A practicing clinician for nearly five decades, Dr. Woolfolk has sought in both his work with patients and his scholarly endeavors to integrate the scientific and humanistic traditions of psychotherapy. He is the author of *The Cure of Souls* and *The Value of Psychotherapy: The Talking Cure in an Age of Clinical Science*, and the coauthor of *Stress, Sanity, and Survival* and *Treating Somatization: A Cognitive Behavioral Approach*.

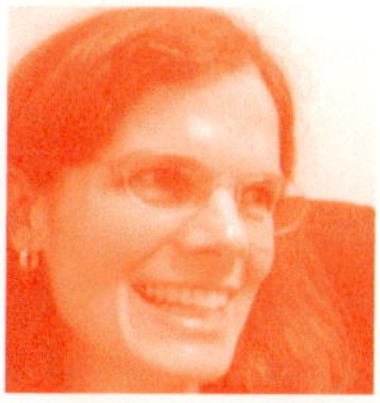

Dr. Allen is Adjunct Associate Professor of Psychiatry at Rutgers Robert Wood Johnson Medical School and a licensed clinical psychologist. She completed her BA at Dartmouth College and graduate degrees (MS and PhD in Clinical Psychology) at Rutgers University. She spent the majority of her academic career developing and studying the efficacy of various treatments for depression, anxiety, and somatic symptom disorders. She received grant funding from the National Institutes of Health and various pharmaceutical companies to study treatments for depression, somatization, and fibromyalgia. Her findings and interpretations of research outcomes have been published in numerous articles, book chapters, and books.

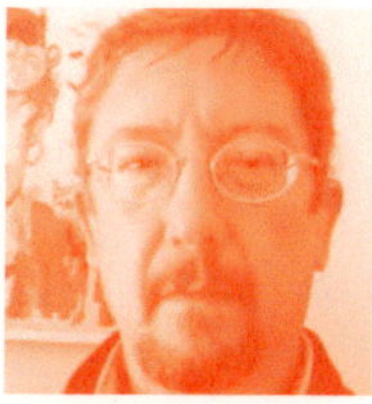

Dr. Federico Durbano received a degree in Medicine and specialized in Psychiatry in Milan. He has had different work experiences in a number of hospitals (Milan "Ospedale Maggiore Policlinico," Treviglio, Melegnano, and Fatebenefratelli), where he achieved significant career milestones. He is now the Director of the Psychiatric Unit in Melzo Hospital—ASST Melegnano e della Martesana—and Vice Director of the Mental Health and Substance Dependence Department at the same ASST. He has had teaching assignments from the University of Milan (Nursing School) and the University of Castellanza (Master in Criminology). He has attended more than 70 local and national congresses and courses as an invited speaker, and has published more than 160 papers in national and international journals and books. He also works as a technical advisor to the court in the field of forensic psychiatry.

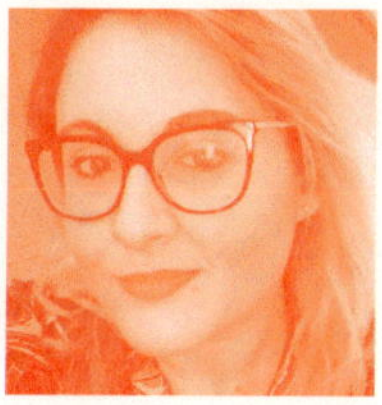

Floriana Irtelli, psychoanalyst, psychotherapist, member of the Italian Society of Psychoanalysis of Relationships, has been lecturing for several years at the Catholic University of the Sacred Heart, Milan, Italy. She has worked at the Fatebenefratelli Hospital, Milan, performing scientific research and clinical activities. She is the coauthor of *A Fresh Look at Anxiety Disorders and Psychopathy: New Updates on an Old Phenomenon*, and has published articles for the *Journal of Affective Disorders, Journal of Research in Psycho-*

therapy, and *Journal of Psychiatric and Mental Health Nursing*. She has participated in numerous conferences, seminars, and congresses, such as the 2015 World Congress of Psycho-Oncology. She is the author of *Illuminarsi di Ben-essere, Familiar-mente, Contemporary Perspectives on Relational Wellness, Psychoanalysis and the Modern Family*, and the editor of *Psychosis, Biopsychosocial and Relational Perspectives.*

Contents

Preface

As the rates of mental illness rise worldwide, it becomes even more vital that the fields that study the etiology and amelioration of mental disorders develop a more complete understanding of the etiology of psychopathology and develop better methods for its amelioration. This collection brings together, from a diverse set of international scientists, a valuable set of perspectives on recent developments in the various areas central to mental health.

Some contributions deal with common emotional disorders, specifically anxiety and affective disturbances. Anxiety will be the leading psychiatric disease in the near future, according to the World Health Organization, bypassing depression. Other contributions give new suggestions on how anxiety and affective disorders influence our daily lives.

In this book, we think that the contributions of clinicians and academics will help in understanding and sharing the "real world" of psychiatry, and we look forward to further developments in this form of knowledge dissemination.

As editors of this volume, we have been aided by the superb staff at IntechOpen. To them we offer our thanks. The dissemination of knowledge without charge to scholars via the internet is an important contribution to the advancement of knowledge. This development is still in its early years, but is destined to have a major impact on all fields of intellectual endeavor.

Robert Woolfolk
Rutgers University,
New Brunswick,
New Jersey, USA

Federico Dubano
Università degli Studi di Milano,
Milano, Italy

Azienda Socio-Sanitaria Territoriale Melegnano e della Martesana,
Melzo Hospital,
Melzo, Italy

Section 1

Psychopathology: An International, Interdisciplinary Perspective

Chapter 1

Introductory Chapter: New Directions in the Study of Psychopathology

Robert L. Woolfolk

1. Introduction

This volume appears at an especially propitious time for psychiatry, clinical psychology, social work, and all the systematic attempts to ameliorate the morbidity and the mortality that is associated with abnormal function of the mind. One can say with conviction that many of the assumptions held by mental health professions for the last half century have come to be challenged and may prove to be false. What do I mean by this?

1. The presumptively atheoretical DSMs, III through V, have not proved to be tools that facilitated scientific progress in the theoretical conceptualization of psychopathology [1]. Nor have they provided clinicians with the kinds of precise diagnostic instruments that would guide treatment. The atheoretical descriptive precision of the DSMs introduces the problem of comorbidity wherein it is rarely the case that single patient will be adequately described by a single diagnosis. This fact greatly compromises the precision of research designs and has led us into a world of polypharmacy that makes the design of pharmacological or psychosocial interventions not only overly complex, but often reduces it to an inductive process of trial and error. Drugs, that in theory should improve depression, sometimes turn out to be more effective with anxiety. Supplementation with atypical anti-psychotics is widely practiced, though with limited empirical evidence.

2. The National Institute of Mental Health already has begun to move away from the approach of the DSMs, which is to define mental disorders based on clusters of symptoms that tend to covary [2]. The approach that may substitute for the DSMs is the putatively more scientific RDoC, or research domain criteria. RDoC is an attempt to return to theory that is structured by basic psychological dimensions: negative valence, positive valence, cognitive processes, social processes, and arousal/regulatory processes.

3. In the U.S. and Europe, the process for approving psychotropic drugs has fostered corruption and poor science. The overstated claims for the efficacy of psychotropic drugs has cast a pall of a field that was in the early 1990s considered on the brink of breakthrough success [3].

At this watershed moment in the mental health sciences, it is a particularly apt time to present an illustrious array of international experts and the scholarship that they bring to central and foundational issues in the field. The topics our author

IntechOpen

addresses range from substance abuse to anxiety, to prenatal factors, to the pathogenic effects of combat. These chapters are grounded in clinical observation and the best research practices. They represent a fascinating array of different perspective appropriate to the beginning of a new era in the mental health sciences.

Author details

Robert L. Woolfolk
Rutgers University, New Brunswick, New Jersey, USA

*Address all correspondence to: rwool@psych.rutgers.edu

References

[1] Hyman SE. Revolution stalled. Science Translational Medicine. 2012;**4**(155cm11):1-4

[2] Insel TR. Next-generational treatments for mental disorders. Science Translational Medicine. 2012;**4**(155ps19):1-9

[3] Wunderink L, Nieboer RM, Wiersma D, Sytema S, Nienhuis FJ. Recovery in remitted first-episode psychosis at 7 years of follow-up of an early dose reduction/discontinuation or maintenance treatment strategy: Long-term follow-up of a 2-year randomized clinical trial. JAMA Psychiatry. 2013;**70**:913-920

Chapter 2

Evidence for Link Between Mental Disorders and in Utero Exposure to Synthetic Hormones: A Long and Crucial History

Marie-Odile Soyer-Gobillard, Laura Gaspari and Charles Sultan

Abstract

Somatic effects of diethylstilbestrol on children exposed in utero have long been recognized. This is not the case for psychiatric disorders, although animal studies provide evidence of somatic and behavioral disorders. Recent studies have reported psychiatric effects of synthetic estrogens on the brain of children exposed in utero as schizophrenia, bipolar disorders, depression, eating disorders, suicides, suicide attempts. Recently, a team of St. Anne's Hospital, Paris (Prof. Krebs, Dr. Kebir) demonstrated the epigenetic mechanism of DES effect on the brain, a specific methylation of two genes playing important roles in neurodevelopment: the ADAM TS9 (control of the formation of reproductive organs and of the fetus's CNS) and the ZFP 57 gene suggested to be associated with psychosis. Progestins used in contraception and in hormone replacement therapy are known to affect the adult brain, but no data on children existed before our recent paper on their effects after in utero exposure. Clinical data were collected from 1934 children of the Association of Patients HHORAGES cohort. Our data show the presence of somatic disorders and a drastic increase of psychiatric disorders among children in utero exposed to progestins. These mental disorders are the same as pathologies provoked by exposure to synthetic estrogens.

Keywords: synthetic estrogens, diethylstilbestrol, ethinyl estradiol, synthetic progestins, mental disorders, in utero exposure

1. Introduction

At the end of the 1990s, somewhere in France, an agricultural engineer, Mr. RA, made the observation that his three children were suffering from various psychic and somatic pathologies, the elder suffering from bilateral cryptorchidism, micropenis, infertility due to azoospermia (no spermatozoa), and schizotypal character; the second from anxiety, depression, and eating disorders (anorexia) coupled with small uterus and ovaries; and the third suffering from schizophrenia and severe depression associated with suicide attempts. He observed also the relationship with the fact that in all three cases, his wife received medical treatment consisting of a synthetic hormone cocktail: diethylstilbestrol (DES), ethinyl estradiol (EE), plus synthetic progestin delay during her three pregnancies after a previous miscarriage. He conducted research in the world literature on the subject and came to the conclusion that not only was one of these products, diethylstilbestrol (DES), already known for its misdeeds but that it continued to be administered in France until 1977/1982. The product, inexpensive to make, was not patented and was manufactured and distributed by many pharmaceutical laboratories. The same goes for EE, which was banned for pregnant women in 1980 but remains the best-selling estrogen in the world because it is part of the contraceptive pill.

In 1998, one of us (MOS-G), concerned by the same kind of problems in her two children who were exposed in utero to the same cocktail of synthetic estrogens, lost her two children after psychiatric illnesses. Following the reading of a "Call to Families" printed in a newspaper, she met Mr. RA, who had gathered around him about 20 French families concerned with their in utero-exposed children suffering from psychiatric illnesses. He wanted to expose his observations and the results of his bibliographic researches at a meeting of patient families collecting observations on the genital malformations of girls exposed in utero to DES. Alas, he was condemned, rejected, and disclaimed by doctors, mostly gynecologists and psychiatrists as well as by associative members. They denied the existence of psychiatric disorders in exposed boys and girls. Discouraged, Mr. RA died shortly afterward. In order to continue his work and regroup the families concerned by the origin of the heavy psychiatric pathologies of their children and despite the taboo surrounding such diseases as psychoses, we gathered several mothers concerned and created the Association of Patients Halt to Artificial Hormones for Pregnancies (HHORAGES), in 2002. This Association which collected more than 1300 French spontaneous testimonies is now registered with the Epidemiology Portal of French National Institute for Medical Research (INSERM) as a French Health Database.

Despite various alerts published in the 1940s, after work on animals proving in particular its carcinogenic effect, and despite the work of Dieckman et al. [1], initiated as early as 1953, demonstrating in a large cohort of pregnant women given diethylstilbetrol (DES), a synthetic estrogen, *versus placebo* that the drug was inefficient in preventing miscarriages or premature births, this product has been widely distributed around the world, sowing a long list of misdeeds. After the discovery of cervicovaginal cancers called "clear cells adenoma (CCAD)" [2] in the "DES girls," DES was banned in the United States for pregnant women in 1971 but only in 1977 in France, where this recommendation disappeared from the "French Vidal book," but DES continued to be prescribed sporadically until 1982. Meanwhile another synthetic estrogen, steroidal, also synthesized on 1938, 17-alpha-ethinyl estradiol (EE), was often added to DES as a cocktail or later as a replacement, sometimes with the addition of synthetic-delay progestin. The idea that prevailed at the time was that women had a hormonal deficit that triggered a miscarriage, whereas now we know that the miscarriage itself causes this deficiency. These products were prescribed not only to women who had miscarriages but also in comfort ("to have beautiful babies," according to an advertising) or even as a "morning after pill" or to cut milk after childbirth. DES and 17-alpha-EE, although belonging to different estrogenic and degrading categories, are, however, bound to the same ER beta-estrogen receptors.

2. Behavioral disorders demonstrated in animals (rats) exposed in utero

Animal studies (on mice and rats) have demonstrated the toxicity of these synthetic estrogens on the offspring, including the cause of behavioral disorders [3–8]. Palanza et al. [3] demonstrated in particular that prenatal exposure to three different synthetic chemicals, DES and two pesticides, DDT and methoxychlor, and its analog, affects the behavior of young suckling mice, showing increased aggression in males (increased numbers of attacks and decreased reaction time before the attack) (**Figure 1**). Doses of DES were 1000 times less than those of DDT and caused much larger aggression responses, demonstrating the considerable effect of DES at very low doses. The treatment period for rodent mothers from day 11 to day 17 of pregnancy was also critical because it represents a key period in the differentiation of the reproductive system and brain development in these rodents in the early stages of pregnancy.

Moreover, injection of 17-alpha-estradiol (EE) in pregnant rats causes not only many abortions in mothers but also anxiety and depression disorders in offspring [4, 5], the synthetic hormone having been administered at the same relative doses as in humans (15 g/kg, 1 per day, versus 19 g/kg, 1 per day). At the cytological level of the brain, an alteration of the anterior part of the hippocampus in young rats exposed to EE in utero has been demonstrated in 2004 [6]. The hippocampus is indeed a part of the brain that contains many estrogen receptors during the prenatal period. Ogiue-Ikeda et al. [7] showed in 2008 that synaptic plasticity can

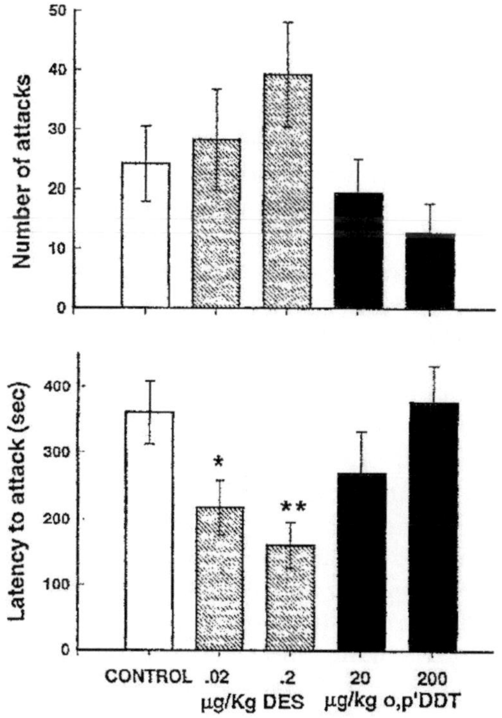

Figure 1.
Measurement of aggressiveness in young male mice after prenatal exposure to diethylstilbestrol (DES) (0.02 and 0.2 µg/kg) [in gray], DDT [20 and 200 µg/kg] [in black], with a control without DES [in white]. There is an increase in the number of attacks and a decrease of the reaction time before the attack although the doses of DES are 1000 times less than those of DDT. According to Palanza et al. [3], with the permission of Elsevier (License No: 2514671323242).

be upset by estrogens or other endocrine disruptors (EDs). Later and unequivocally, Newbold demonstrated the validity of the rodent model transposed to humans [8].

3. Behavioral disorders, psychoses, and depression demonstrated in humans after in utero exposure to DES/EE

In humans, the work concerning the appearance of behavioral disorders in children after in utero exposure to synthetic hormones is less numerous, but as early as 1977, June Reinisch [9] published in Nature that prenatal exposure to estrogen and/or synthetic progestins could affect the personality of exposed children. More recently, in 2012, Kebir and Krebs [10] have analyzed several epidemiological studies concerning the effects of DES on exposed children in utero and the occurrence of psychiatric disorders in these children. Their analysis shows that only three large epidemiological studies on the effects of DES were performed in 1952–1953 (followed up in 1983), in 2007, and in 2010. The first study (double-blinded) that supports the hypothesis of a link between psychiatric disorders and prenatal exposure to DES was performed by Vessey et al., in 1983 [11], from a clinical trial that had been performed 30 years earlier in 1953 in London by Dieckman et al., on 700 women treated with DES versus 700 subjected to a placebo [1]. A doubling of depression and anxiety disorders has been demonstrated in the population exposed in utero. The second, published in 2007 and conducted by Verdoux et al. [12], from a cohort of women from the Mutuelle (Health) de l'Education Nationale (MGEN) concludes that there are no significant links between exposure to DES, suicides, and/or psychiatric consultations or hospitalizations. A detailed analysis later, however, revealed a number of biases in this study [13]. The most recent Nurses' Health Study was conducted by O'Reilly et al., 2010 [14], from 76,240 American women among whom 1612 women were exposed to DES in utero. The statistical analysis shows that the latter experienced an increase in depressive and anxiety disorders by a factor of 1.3. Kebir and Krebs [10] emphasized the limitations of such epidemiological studies and noted in particular that, apart from depression and anxiety, other psychiatric disorders have not been studied. Postadolescence behavioral disturbances reported for these two estrogens in exposed children were depression [15, 16], anxiety [1, 11, 17], schizophrenia-like behavior [18, 19], anorexia, and bulimia nervosa [20]. All these observations were synthesized by Pillard et al. [16] and Giusti [21]. On 1987, Katz et al. [18] described the case of four male adults prenatally exposed to DES. It is in late adolescence that they develop psychotic disorders requiring neuroleptic treatment even though they have no family history of this type. He then hypothesizes that there may be a causal relationship between disruptions in neurodevelopment related to DES and the subsequent onset of psychotic disorders. Pillard et al. [16] showed that the frequency of recurrent major depressive episodes is significantly higher in the DES-exposed than in their unexposed siblings, which was confirmed in 2010 in the large cohort of DES girls by O'Reilly et al. [14].

Investigation of the causal link between exposure to these synthetic hormones in utero and severe psychotic disorders such as schizophrenia, bipolar disorders with or without eating disorders, and schizoaffective disorders, occurring in post-adolescence in exposed children, was made possible thanks to the families of the Association HHORAGES. Our database, constituted by these spontaneous families' testimonies, is based on responses to a detailed questionnaire, written by doctors and researchers and accepted by the CNIL (French Center for the Protection of Data Processing and Freedom). Our first global analysis (2004–2005 data) was based on 967 pregnancies from 470 mothers in collaboration between 2 of us (MOS-G/CS) of us (CS). The first results as well as the family questionnaires were detailed in 2012 in the chapter published in 2012 by InTech "Behavioral and Somatic Disorders in Children Exposed In Utero to Synthetic Hormones" [13] in which we detailed somatic and psychiatric disorders, associated or not, in the exposed children of our cohort.

We have conducted a more recent analysis (2016) [22, 23] based on 1182 pregnancies from 529 mothers (**Figure 2**).

Among the 740 (20 stillborn) exposed children, 603 (exposed) +16 post-DES (born without exposure but after a previous exposed pregnancy) are suffering from psychiatric disorders. The prevalence of the psychiatric disorders in comparison with the general population shows a dramatic increase (**Table 1**).

We were also interested by the effects on the brain of synthetic progestins on in utero-exposed children of our cohort (**Figures 3** and **4**). Currently, there is no research on these effects of in utero exposure of children to progestins given alone during pregnancy. Our recent observations [24, 25] were collected from 1200 families of the HHORAGES cohort, that is, 1934 children using always the same detailed questionnaire [13]. As previously shown, most families of our cohort had children exposed to estrogens or to estro-progestins, but only 46 families (115 children) had at least 1 child exposed to 1 or more progestins prescribed alone and representing 62 in utero-exposed children. Thirty-five children were post-exposed (**Figure 3**). The prescribed progestins were 17-α-hydroxyprogesterone caproate (synthetic progestin, SP) against total indication in 2000 but reauthorized in 2011, 17-α-hydroxyprogesterone heptanoate (SP) against total indication in 2002, and chlormadinone acetate (SP), derived from hydroxyprogesterone, against total indication in 1970.

Among the 62 exposed children (22 girls and 40 boys), 49 presented psychiatric disorders, 6 presented somatic disorders only, and 7 did not present any disorder. Only 1 post-exposed presented psychiatric disorder, while 34 other post-exposed did not present any disorder.

Among the 49 children affected by psychiatric disorders, 3 boys and 7 girls presented both somatic disorders in addition to psychiatric ones: boys (3), hypospadias (1), no urinary meatus (1), bilateral cryptorchidia, and sexual ambiguity (1) and girls (7), hormonal sterility (2), hirsutism and enuresis (1), enuresis (1), hirsutism (1), hermaphrodism (1, operated), and sexual ambiguity and tight

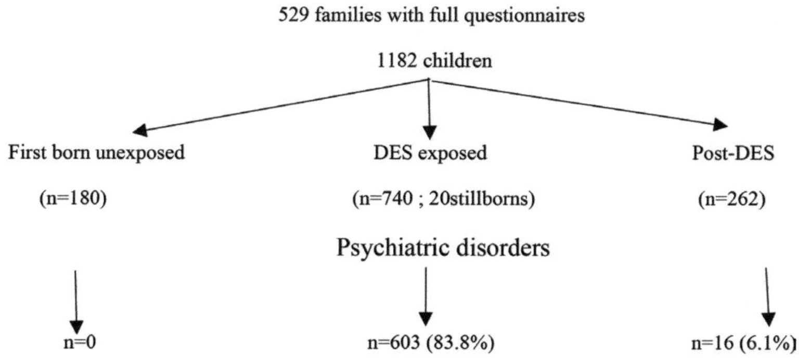

Figure 2.
Total number of psychological/psychiatric disorders among the 982 (1002 total with 20 stillborns) DES-exposed and post-DES unexposed children. First-born children (intrafamilial control) unexposed are not ill.

	Group 1	Group 2	Group 3	
	First-born pre-DES	DES-exposed	Post-DES	General population
	n = 180	n = 740-20	n = 262	
Behavioral disorders	0%	n = 109 (15.1%)	n = 1 (0.4%)	3%
Schizophrenia	0%	n = 165 (22.9%)	n = 6 (2.3%)	1%
Eating disorders	0%	n = 81 (11.3%)	n = 2 (0.8%)	1.6%
Depression				
Bipolar disorders, anxiety	0%	n = 248 (34.4%)	n = 9 (3.4%)	6.3%
Suicide attempts	0%	n = 612 (85%)	n = 30 (11.5%)	0.3%
Death	0%	n = 32 (4.4%)	n = 1 (0.4%)	0.02%

Table 1.
Prevalences of the psychological and/or psychiatric disorders in in utero-exposed children to DES and/or EE and comparison with the general population [23].

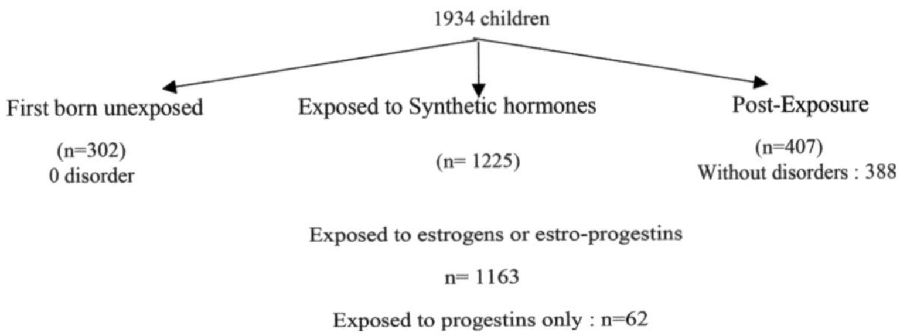

Figure 3.
Total HHORAGES cohort of 1934 children in which 3 groups can be observed.

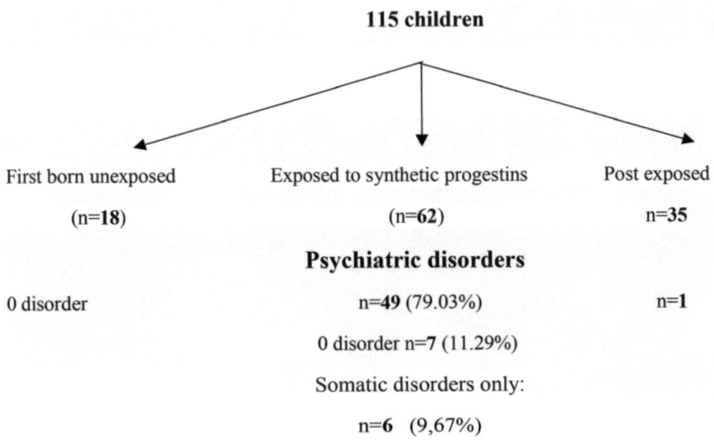

Figure 4.
Division of the 115 children of the 46 "progestins" families: first-born unexposed, in utero exposed, and post exposed, that is, born after a previous exposed pregnancy.

urethra (1). Among the six exposed children suffering from somatic disorders "only," we observed for boys (four) mega bilateral ureter (one grandchild), unilateral cryptorchidia (one), hypospadias with numerous interventions of

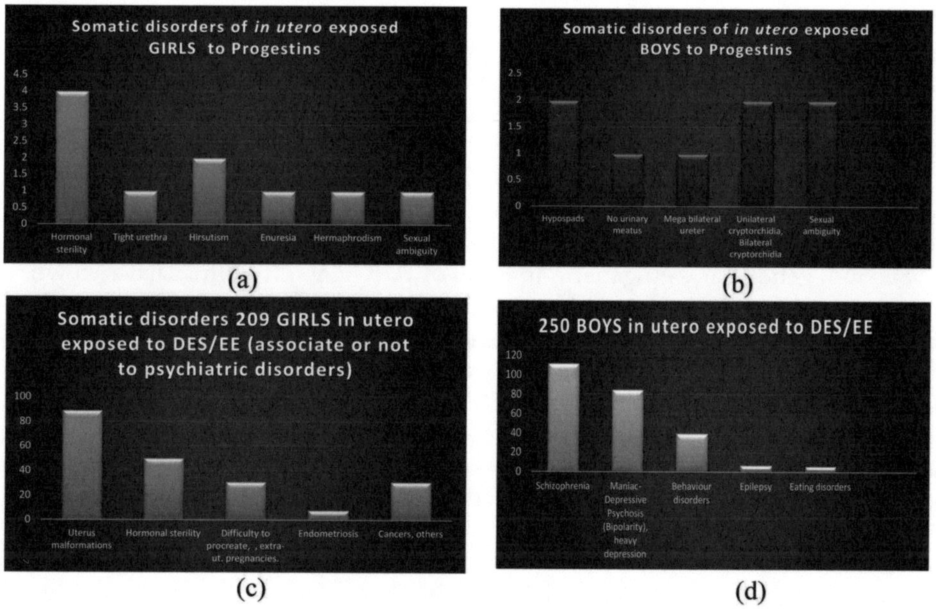

Figure 5.
Comparative diagrams representing psychiatric disorder cases presented, respectively, by girls (a, c) and boys (b, d) exposed either to synthetic estrogens diethylstilbestrol (DES) and ethinyl estradiol (EE) (c, d) or to synthetic progestins (a, b).

reconstruction (one grandchild), and sexual ambiguity (one) and for girls (two) hormonal sterility (two).

As shown in **Figure 5**, a comparison of synthetic estrogen and progestin exposures for girls and boys demonstrates that psychiatric disorders were of the same nature for progestin exposure as those observed after exposure to synthetic estrogens, that is, behavioral disorders = 2, eating disorders = 2, schizophrenia = 29, depression, bipolar disorders = 16, suicides attempts = 7 series, and death = 1. The percentage of suicide attempts (11.29%) and death after suicide (1.6%) is proportionately lower after exposure to progestins than after exposure to synthetic estrogens.

4. An epigenetic mechanism

Search for the molecular basis of the causal link between in utero, exposure to synthetic hormones and the appearance of psychoses as schizophrenia or bipolar disorder in children exposed in utero, has been achieved thanks to the partnership that unites HHORAGES Patients' Association with the INSERM team of molecular psychiatrist Pr. MO Krebs (St. Anne's Hospital, Paris, France, UMR S 894), which began in 2007. "It would have been 'crazy' to miss the problem posed by the Association Hhorages to establish a causal link between taking artificial hormone (s) during pregnancy and appearance of psychiatric disorders of the type psychotic in exposed children, because diethylstilbestrol (Distilbene® or DES) has been given over a limited period of time and people who have taken this molecule are still there to testify. This is a case study that should not be missed" said Dr. Kebir (Center for Psychiatry and Neuroscience, UMR S 894), manager of these researches as part of the Krebs' team.

First, to document in utero exposure to synthetic estrogens, Kebir and Krebs [10] were able to analyze from our data a small number of family records that occurred in HHORAGES testimonies and studied a cohort of 472 exposed subjects. They account for 46.7% of mood disorders, 22.9% of psychotic disorders, 6.6% of anxiety disorders, 11% of eating disorders, and 12.7% of others, which confirms their previous observations published on 2009 and 2010 at the seventh and eighth Congress of the Encephalon in Paris [26, 27] on 43 exposed children highlighting clinical pictures with atypical associations.

Second, genetic and epigenetic analyses of HHORAGES siblings have shown in patients suffering from psychotic disorders and exposed in utero to DES and/or EE that this prenatal exposure is associated with epigenetic processes. Starting from the fact that psychiatric diseases develop from a brain dysfunction during neurodevelopment, and knowing that DES and EE are synthetic hormones (estrogens), endocrine disruptors, and confirming from the HHORAGES data numerous cases of heavy psychiatric disorders in children exposed, the Krebs'team in association with HHORAGES designed 10 years ago, in 2007, a research project Partnership Citizen Institution for Research and Innovation (PICRI), funded by the Ile de France Region, net by the French National REsearch Agency (ANR), that developed the hypothesis that the DES administered during pregnancies could be an environmental risk factor for the development of psychiatric disorders in impregnated children: the epigenome of the foetus could have been modified by in utero exposure to synthetic estrogens. The PICRI project was titled "Influence of hormonal treatments on brain development during pregnancy: study of phenotypic, behavioral and biological changes in informative families." The families of HHORAGES were called to perform peripheral blood sampling after thorough questioning. Many families volunteered to participate in the research: 31 families were selected, satisfying the rigorous inclusion criteria desired. Many more families had come forward during this study, but they could not be included because the psychotic patient refused to come to St. Anne's Hospital for blood sampling. In the selected families, total siblings were composed of first-born unexposed children, exposed children, and post-exposed children, with first-born unexposed serving as intrafamilial control. For the exploration of their epigenome, 485,000 cytosines by genome were studied and analyzed, representing an immense work. To complete this study, a cohort of young adolescents with relational, emotional, and social difficulties was followed for 6 months, some of whom had developed schizophrenic-type psychosis in these 6 months, although not exposed to DES. A comparison of their methylome, analyzed before and after the onset of the disease, was performed. In this study [28], authors reported a global methylation of the psychotic patient genome.

After the analysis of the whole methylome of the selected HHORAGES cohort, the team of Krebs-Kebir highlighted differential specific methylated regions (DMR): in the zinc finger protein 57 gene ZFP57 and in the ADAM TS9gene and in young psychotic patients exposed in utero to DES/EE [29, 30]. In this work, the authors observed that in exposed individuals, ZFP57 gene methylation may be associated with their psychosis. The ZFP57 gene (located on chromosome 6) is expressed very early in development. It is a transcription regulator, directly related to the phenomenon of methylation and neurodevelopment [31]. The ADAM TS9 gene is implicated in the control of organ shape, especially in the development and function of the uterus and reproductive organs [32] which are often abnormal after in utero DES exposure as well as in the control of the CNS development [33] and in several kinds of cancers [34].

5. Discussion and conclusion

Very few studies have investigated the impact of prenatal exposure to DES and EE on psychiatric outcome. Animal studies on rats or mice allowed us to hypothesize that estrogenic hormones induce neurodevelopmental disturbances in exposed human subjects and may potentially mediate an increased risk of behavioral and psychiatric disorders. Our data therefore strongly suggest that DES/EE exposure during pregnancy is associated with high incidence of behavioral and/or psychiatric disorders. They illustrate a higher risk of schizophrenia, as this disease was 17 times more prevalent than in the general population, with sons being more affected than DES daughters. Regarding the existence of eating disorders (bulimia, anorexia), it should be noted that girls are much more affected than boys, and we often observed the association of eating disorders with bipolarity (manic-depressive disorders), anxiety, and depression. With regard to suicides, our work clearly demonstrates a drastically increased risk of suicide attempts (65.4% versus 0 in the unexposed controls and 0.25% in the general population) and suicides (3.4% versus 0 in the unexposed controls and 0.02% in the general population). It could be noted that, as in the general population, DES sons commit more suicides than DES daughters and the inverse for suicide attempts. Moreover, our data reveal that 50% of the sons who committed suicide suffered from schizophrenia. Psychiatric studies in general have shown that the percentage of suicides is generally higher in individuals with psychiatric disorders than in the general population. But to our knowledge, there is no information or specific studies concerning this association in the context of DES exposure. Sixteen subjects in Group 3 (post-DES children) (**Figure 2** and **Table 1**) had diagnosed psychiatric disorders. An explanation for this finding might be that DES, being a very lipophilic synthetic estrogen, remains in the mothers' fat after estrogenic impregnation in a previous pregnancy and is then released through the placental barrier during the next gestation.

No work had been reported on the impact of in utero exposure to synthetic progestin hormones administered alone on the occurrence of psychiatric disorders in exposed children before our first presentation in the European Congress of Gynecology in 2017 [24]. For the first time, we described psychiatric disorders that can affect children exposed in utero to progestins. Previously, and during many years, synthetic progestogens were not considered as dangerous during pregnancy or during replacement or contraceptive treatment. Moreover, they have been suggested to exert neuroprotective effects in several animal models of neurological disease [35]. Negative mood symptoms have been reported by Andreen et al. [36] in some women as a result of progesterone during the luteal phase of menstrual cycles. This is believed to be mediated via the action of allopregnanolone on the GABA-A system. A reduction of allopregnanolone circulating levels that correlates to depressive symptoms has been recently reported [37], and conversely, healthy women reported increased anxiety and mood disorders after long-acting subdermal implant of progestogens. In a group of 236 schizophrenic patients at onset, an elevated concentration of progesterone has been found, and authors suggested that steroid hormones may influence brain function, underlying schizophrenia, and major depressive disorders [38]. Moreover, Buoli et al. (2016) found high DHAS levels in patients with a history of psychotic symptoms, suggesting a role of steroids in the etiology of psychosis and mood disorders [39]. Progestins are known to induce GABA receptor activity/neural activation before birth; it is likely that a GABAergic system could contribute to schizophrenia, anxiety, depression, panic disorders, epilepsy, autism, and others [40]. Although some progestins have been banned from the market, others are not: our data demonstrated that caution should be taken with regard to the use of these progestins during pregnancy and even outside these periods (contraception or hormone replacement therapy).

The brain is a very vulnerable organ because its development covers a very broad period extending from the early prenatal stage (third week of pregnancy) to end around the age of 20. During its development, there are times when its vulnerability is even greater than others; these periods are called "shooting windows," during which the environment can impact the normal process of development. Abdolmaleky et al. [41] as early as 2005 had developed the hypothesis that gene-environment modulations could be performed via DNA methylations. Krebs' team put forward the hypothesis that DES-induced changes in epigenetic background and alteration of DNA functioning (methylations) could be significant factors to demonstrate a possible origin of psychotic disorders and a link with in utero DES exposure of the children suffering from these illnesses [29, 30].

Numerous studies have shown that, for example, in the rat, early maternal separation or the fact of causing significant stress to the mother changes the methylation signals of certain genes of the rat directly related to the regulation of anxiety. It has also been discovered that the proper environment for changing the methylation signals may be chemical. This is the case of DES recognized by the scientific community as an endocrine disruptor and banned for pregnant women. This change in the level of methylation caused in utero by DES has been demonstrated for urogenital malformations of girls and boys as well as for cancers. On 2015, Harlid et al. published in a pioneer work the first study for evaluation of possible effects of in utero DES exposure on genome-wide DNA methylation in humans [42]. They studied whole blood DNA methylation in 100 40–59-year-old women reporting in utero exposure, compared to 100 unexposed women. They did not find any differential methylation, but the DMR approach was not used in their recent work (2015). On the other hand, in 2017 Rivollier et al. [30] described specific differential methylated regions (DMR) on two genes implicated in neurodevelopment (ZFP57 and ADAMTS9). Surprisingly, they cautiously claim that these DMR are "supposedly" associated with prenatal exposure to DES in young psychotic patients in utero exposed to DES/EE. Nevertheless, these modifications of methylation are really specific because they do not exist in the methylome of young psychotic patients not exposed to DES [28] in which global methylation of the genome was observed. Moreover authors have compared exposed subjects to their unexposed siblings which do not present these specific methylations although they shared environmental and genetic factors.

The citizen work carried out between the French HHORAGES Patient Association and two major medical research laboratories has provided convincing scientific results: (1) on the detection and confirmation of the existence of psychiatric disorders (accompanied or not of somatic disorders) in children exposed in utero to synthetic hormones and (2) on the mechanisms of action of these synthetic hormones administered to pregnant mothers on the brain of their offspring. The effects of these endocrine disruptors in humans through what is becoming a public health scandal, denied for a long time by doctors, especially psychiatrists, scientists, and specialized journalists, are thus better known. The fact that these synthetic products do not degrade in the human body in the same way as the natural hormones [13] and act on the functioning of genes implicated in neurodevelopment during the fetal life, following an epigenetic mechanism, is a real time bomb. Indeed, this mechanism induces a transgenerational effect already partially demonstrated in the HHORAGES cohort at the third-generation level for hypospadias, a specific genital malformation. So far, only a few third-generation children suffering psychiatric illness are documented in the HHORAGES testimonies. This is understandable because third-generation exposed children are still too young (excepted in some cases) to present psychiatric disorders as schizophrenia which is not the case for hypospadias that are detectable from birth in male children and grandchildren [43]. In contrast, psychiatric disorders usually appear in postadolescence, 18–20 years, and sometimes later.

Acknowledgements

Mr. René Alexandre, Dr. Henri Pézerat, Pfr. Jean Caston, Mr. Michel Datry, and Dr. Charles Zelwer worked tirelessly to demonstrate the harmful role of the endocrine disruptors and in particular of synthetic hormones; before passing away: we shall never forget their efficient help. This work could not continue without the daily ongoing support of the HHORAGES board especially Mrs. Geneviève A., Mauricette P., Yette B., Annie R., Aimée I., Sylvette C., Denise H., Marie-Noelle P., and Pierre D. We acknowledge Mr. André Cicolella, president of the French Environment-Health network (RES), for his constant support. We are very grateful to Pfr. Michael Dolan, professor at the University of Massachusetts, Amherst (USA), for his help and critical reading during the preparation of the manuscript.

Notes

Association HHORAGES-France is registered on the Epidemiological Portal of French Health Databases INSERM (French National Institute for Medical Research) and AVIESAN (National Alliance for Life Sciences and Health) (epidemiologie-france.aviesan.fr).

Disclaimer

The authors declare they have no competitive financial interests; the finances of HHORAGES-France association come exclusively from the donations of families and of sympathetic individuals.

Author Biography

Marie-Odile Soyer-Gobillard: National Center for Scientific Research (CNRS), Sorbonne University, P. and M. Curie University, Paris 6, and HHORAGES Association (Halt to Artificial Hormones for Pregnancies), The Priory of Baillon, F-95270 Asnieres sur Oise, France. Email: elido66@orange.fr. Doctor of Science (Cell Biology), Honorary Emeritus Research Director at CNRS, laureate of several scientific awards, and author of more than 150 publications in peer-reviewed scientific journals. Former Director of the Department of Cellular and Molecular Biology (UMR 796 "Models in Cell and Evolutive Biology") at the Arago Laboratory (Paris 6 University) and expert at the National Agency for Research (ANR). National president of HHORAGES, France (Stop to Artificial Hormones for Pregnancy) and president of its Scientific Council. Member of the Clinical Projects Reviewers Committee, INSERM, Paris.

Charles Sultan: Unité d'endocrinologie et gynécologie pédiatrique, Hôpital Arnaud-de-Villeneuve, CHU de Montpellier, 34295 Montpellier Cedex 5, France. Email: c-sultan@chu-montpellier.fr

Laura Gaspari: Unité d'endocrinologie et gynécologie pédiatrique, Hôpital Arnaud-de-Villeneuve, CHU de Montpellier, 34295 Montpellier Cedex 5, France. Email: dr.lauragaspari@gmail.com

Author details

Marie-Odile Soyer-Gobillard[1,2*], Laura Gaspari[3] and Charles Sultan[3]

1 National Center for Scientific Research (CNRS), Sorbonne University, P. and M. Curie, Paris, France

2 National President of HHORAGES Association (Halt to Artificial Hormones for Pregnancies), The Priory of Baillon, Asnières sur Oise, France

3 Unité d'endocrinologie et de gynécologie pédiatrique, Hôpital Arnaud-de-Villeneuve, CHU de Montpellier, Montpellier, France

*Address all correspondence to: elido66@orange.fr

References

[1] Dieckman WJ, Davis ME, Rynkiewicz LM, Pottinger RE. Does the administration of diethylstilbestrol during pregnancy have therapeutic value? American Journal of Obstetrics and Gynaecology. 1953;**66**:1062-1081

[2] Herbst AL, Ulfelder H, Poskanzer DC. Adenocarcinoma of the vagina. Association of maternal stilbestrol therapy with tumor appearance in young women. New England Journal of Medicine. 1971;**284**(15):878-881

[3] Palanza P, Morellini F, Parmigiani S, Vom Saal FS. Prenatal exposure to endocrine disrupting chemicals: effects on behavioral development. Neuroscience and Biobehavioral Reviews. 1999;**23**:1011-1027

[4] Dugard ML, Tremblay-Leveau H, Mellier D, Caston J. Prenatal exposure to ethinylestradiol elicits behavioural abnormalities in the rat. Developmental Brain Research. 2001;**129**:189-199

[5] Arabo A, Lefebvre M, Fermanel M, Caston J. Administration of 17-alphaethinylestradiol during pregnancy elicits modifications of maternal behaviour and emotional alteration of the offspring in the rat. Developmental Brain Research. 2005;**156**:93-103

[6] Sandner G, Barbosa Silva MJ, Angst J, Knobloch JM, Danion JM. Prenatal exposure of Long-Evans rats to 17alpha-ethinylestradiol modifies neither latent inhibition nor prepulse inhibition of the statle reflex but elicits minor deficiency in exploratory behaviour. Developmental Brain Research. 2004;**152**:177-187

[7] Ogiue-Ikeda M, Tanabe N, Mukai H, Hojo Y, Murakami G, Tsurugizawa T, et al. Rapid modulation of synaptic plasticity by estrogens as well as endocrine disrupters in hippocampal neurons. Brain Research Reviews. 2008;**57**(2):363-375. DOI: 10.1016/j.brainresrev.2007.06.010 PMID: 17822775

[8] Newbold RR. Lessons learned from perinatal exposure to diethylstilbestrol. Toxicology and Applied Pharmacology. 2004;**199**:142-150

[9] Reinisch JM. Prenatal exposure of human foetuses to synthetic progestin and oestrogen affects personality. Nature. 1977;**266**:561-562

[10] Kebir O, Krebs MO. Diethylstilbestrol and risk of psychiatric disorders: A critical review and new insights. The World Journal of Biological Psychiatry. 2012;**13**(2):84-95

[11] Vessey MP, Faiweather DV, Norman-Smith B, Buckley J. A randomized double-blind controlled trial of the value of stilboestrol therapy in pregnancy: long term follow-up of mothers and their offspring. BJOG: An International Journal of Obstetrics & Gynaecology. 1983;**90**:1007-1017

[12] Verdoux H, Ropers J, Costagliola D, Clavel-Chapelon F, Paoletti X. Serious psychiatric outcome of subjects prenatally exposed to diethylstilbestrol in the E3N cohort study. Psychological Medicine. 2007;**37**:1315-1322

[13] Soyer-Gobillard MO, Sultan C. Behavioral and Somatic Disorders in Children exposed *in utero* to Synthetic Hormones : a Testimony-Case Study in a French Family Troop. In: Magdeldin S, editor. State of the Art of Therapeutic Endocrinology. Niigata University, Japan: InTech; 2012. pp. 67-86

[14] O'Reilly EJ, Mirzaei F, Forman MR, Ascherio A. Diethylstilbestrol exposure in utero and depression in women. American Journal of Epidemiology. 2010;**171**:876-882

[15] Ehrhardt AA, Feldman JF, Rosen LR, Meyer-Bahlburg R, Gruen NP, Veridiano NP, et al. Psychopathology in prenatally DES-exposed females: current and lifetime adjustment. Psychosomatic Medicine. 1987;**49**:183-196

[16] Pillard RC, Rosen H, Meyer-Bahlburg JD, Weinrich JF, Feldman JF, Gruen R, et al. Psychopathology and social functioning in men prenatally exposed to diethylstilbestrol (DES). Psychosomatic Medicine. 1993;**55**:485-491

[17] Saunders G. Physical and psychological problems associated with exposure to diethylstilbestrol (DES). Hospital & Community Psychiatry. 1988;**39**:73-77

[18] Katz DL, Frankenburg FR, Frances R, Benowitz LI, Gilbert JM. Psychosis and prenatal exposure to diethylstilbestrol. The Journal of Nervous and Mental Disease. 1987;**175**:306-308

[19] Verdoux H. Quelles sont les conséquences psychiatriques de l'exposition intra-utérine au diethylstilbestrol (DES)? Annales Médico-Psychologiques. 2000;**158**:105-117

[20] Geary N. The effect of estrogen on appetite. Medscape Women's Health. 1998;**3**(10):3

[21] Giusti RM, Iwamoto K, Hatch E. Diethylstilbestrol revisited: A review of the long term health effects. Annals of Internal Medicine. 1995;**122**:778-788

[22] Soyer-Gobillard MO, Paris F, Gaspari L, Courtet Ph, Sultan Ch. Endocrine disruptors (ED) and psychiatric disorders in children exposed *in utero*: Evidence from a French cohort of 1002 prenatally exposed children and the example of diethylstilbestrol (DES) as a model for ED study. 2nd PARIS Workshop on Endocrine Disruptors: Effects on Wildlife and Human Health. Paris (Institut Pasteur), 21-22 Janvier 2016; 2016

[23] Soyer-Gobillard MO, Gaspari-Sultan L, Paris F, Courtet P, Sultan C. Association between foetal DES-exposure and psychiatric disorders in adolescence/adulthood: evidence from a French cohort of 1002 prenatally exposed children. Gynecological Endocrinology. 2016;**32**(1):25-29. DOI: 10.3109/09513590.2015.1063604

[24] Soyer-Gobillard MO, Gaspari-Sultan L, Paris F, Courtet Ph, Sultan Ch. Neurodevelopmental disorders in children exposed *in utero* to progestin treatment: study of a cohort of 95 children from the HHORAGES Association. 12è Congress of the European Society of Gynecology, Barcelona, 18-21 October 2017; 2017

[25] Soyer-Gobillard MO, Gaspari-Sultan L, Paris F, Courtet Ph, Puillandre M, Sultan Ch. Neurodevelopmental disorders in children exposed *in utero* to synthetic Progestins: Analysis from the national cohort of the Hhorages Association. Just accepted by Gynecological Endocrinology. https://doi.org/10.1080/09513590.2018.1512968

[26] Roblin J, Chayet M, Bon Saint Come M, Kebir O, Bannour S, Guedj F, Krebs M-O. Troubles psychiatriques et exposition *in utero* aux hormones de synthèse: Etude d'une série de cas. 7ème Congrès de l'Encéphale, Paris. 2009, 22-24-01, PO 010

[27] Kebir O, Chayet M, Gorsane M-A, Ben Jemaa N, Krebs M-O. Exposition durant la grossesse aux hormones de synthèse et augmentation du risque des troubles psychiatriques: revue critique. 8ème Congrès de l'Encéphale, Paris. 2010;**36**:3-9. PO. 001

[28] Kebir O, Chaumette B, Rivollier F, Miozzo F, Lemieux Perreault LP,

Barhdadi A, et al. Methylomic changes during conversion to psychosis. Molecular Psychiatry. 2016:1-7. DOI: 10.1038/mp.2016.53

[29] Rivollier F, Kebir O, Chaumette B, Krebs MO. Methylomic changes in individuals with psychosis and prenatally exposed to Diethylstilbestrol. Schizophrenia International Research Society Conference, npj Schizophrenia 2016, 16009, PO S202

[30] Rivollier F, Chaumette B, Bendjemaa N, Chayet M, Millet B, Jaafari N, et al. Methylomic changes in individuals with psychosis, prenatally exposed to endocrine disrupting compounds: Lessons from diethylstilbestrol. PLoS One. 2017;**12**(4):e0174783, 10.1371/journal.pone.0174783

[31] Quenneville S, Verde G, Corsinotti A, Kapopoulou A, Jakobsson J, Offner S, et al. In embryonic stem cells, ZFP57/KAP1 recognize a methylated hexanucleotide to affect chromatin and DNA methylation of imprinting control regions. Molecular Cell. 2011;**44**(3): 361-372. DOI: 10.1016/j.molcel.2011.08.032. PMID: 22055183

[32] Mittaz L, Russell DL, Wilson T, Brasted M, Tkalcevic J, Salamonsen LA, et al. Adamts-1 is essential for the development and function of the urogenital system. Biology of Reproduction. 2004 Apr;**70**(4):1096-1105. DOI: 10.1095/biolreprod.103.023911. PMID: 14668204

[33] Lemarchant S, Pruvost M, Montaner J, Emery E, Vivien D, Kanninen K, et al. ADAMTS proteoglycanases in the physiological and pathological central nervous system. Journal of Neuroinflammation. 2013;**10**:133. DOI: 10.1186/1742-2094-10-133. PMID: 24176075

[34] Zhang C, Shao Y, Zhang W, Wu Q, Yang H, Zhong Q, et al. High-resolution melting analysis of ADAMTS9 methylation levels in gastric, colorectal, and pancreatic cancers. Cancer Genetics and Cytogenetics. 2010 Jan 1;**196**(1):38-44. DOI: 10.1016/j.cancergencyto.2009.08.016. PMID: 19963134 37

[35] Melcangi RC, Giatti S, Calabrese D, Pesaresi M, Cermenati G, Mitro N, et al. Levels and actions of progesterone and its metabolites in the nervous system during physiological and pathological conditions. Progress in Neurobiology. 2014;**113**(2):56-69

[36] Andreen L, Nyberg S, Turkmen S, van Wingen G, Fernandez G, Bäckström T. Sex steroid induced negative mood may be explained by the paradoxical effect mediated by GABAA modulators. Psychoneuroendocrinology. 2009;**34**:1121-1132

[37] Slopien R, Pluchino N, Warenik-Szymankiewicz A, Sajdak S, Luisi M, Drakopoulos P, et al. Correlation between allopregnanolone levels and depressive symptoms during late menopausal transition and early postmenopause. Gynecological Endocrinology. 2018;**34**(2):144-147

[38] Guest PC, Schwarz E, Krishnamurthy D, Harris LW, Leweke FM, Rothermundt M, et al. Altered levels of circulating insulin and other neuroendocrine hormones associated with the onset of schizophrenia. Psychoneuroendocrinology. 2011;**36**(7):1092-1096

[39] Buoli M, Caldiroli A, Serati M, Grassi S, Altamura AC. Sex Steroids and Major Psychoses: Which Role for DHEA-S and Progesterone? Neuropsychobiology. 2016;**73**:178-183

[40] Schmidt MJ, Mirnics K. Neurodevelopment, GABA System dysfunction, and schizophrenia.

Neuropsychopharmacology Reviews. 2014:1-17

[41] Abdolmaleky HM, Smith CL, Faraone SV, Shafa R, Stone W, Glatt SJ, et al. Methylomics in psychiatry: modulation of gene–environment interactions may be through DNA methylation. American Journal of Medical Genetics. Part B, Neuropsychiatric Genetics. 2004;**127**:51-59

[42] Harlid S, Xu Z, Panduri V, D'Aloisio AA, DeRoo LA, Sandler DP, et al. In utero exposure to diethylstilbestrol and blood DNA methylation in women ages 40-59 years from the sister study. PLoS One. 2015;**10**(3):e0118757. DOI: 10.1371/journal.pone.0118757. PMID: 25751399

[43] Kalfa N, Paris F, Soyer-Gobillard MO, Daures JP, Sultan C. Incidence of hypospadias in grandsons of DES-exposed women during pregnancy: a multigenerational national cohort study. Fertiity and Sterility. 2011;**95**(8):2574-2577

Chapter 3

Cocaine and Its Variations in Forms of Presentation and Addiction

Antonio Gomes de Castro Neto, Magda da Silva Figueiroa, Renata Barreto Fernandes de Almeida, Rossana Carla Rameh-de-Albuquerque, Iandê dos Santos Gomes de Moura and Solange Aparecida Nappo

Abstract

This chapter intends to show cocaine variations in its forms of presentation, chemical forms, pharmacology, use forms, and contexts of use to understand how these factors can influence drug addiction. Furthermore, a discussion on the most expected psychoactive effects will take place during this chapter, based on different forms of use, treatment possibilities, and possible harm reduction strategies. Above all, the discussion considers the recursive movement of people who abuse the drug or became dependent. Therefore, the authors will discourse about these aspects using some singular and illustrative cases, from the biographical trajectory of people in their contexts related to the substance use, aborting the recursive movement of the drug user.

Keywords: cocaine, molecular forms, forms of presentation, addiction, treatment

1. Introduction

Cocaine is one of the most consumed illicit drugs in the world. It is estimated that 17.1 million people in the world use this substance [1]. The drug is a tropane alkaloid found in leaves of coca plant (*Erythroxylum coca* L.), which only grows in Andean countries [2]. From dry leaves of coca plant is produced the cocaine paste. This product has a high cocaine concentration and can be consumed as a drug or used for the production of many cocaine derivatives [3, 4].

There are many cocaine forms of presentation. Variations in these forms are due to changes in chemical form of the cocaine molecule and also in the way how the drug is consumed. Cocaine molecule can be in molecular or salt form. Both chemical forms have different physical-chemistry properties, which influence the way how the drug will be self-administrated and consequently metabolized by the organism [5].

The drug has a stimulating action in the organism with potential to cause addiction [6]. Cocaine is one of the main substances that can cause more physical damage and chemical dependence on someone [7]. Intensity of effects, dependence, and craving are strongly influenced by the way in which the drug is self-administered.

Compulsive use, besides chemical dependence, can make people susceptible to health problems and affect interpersonal relationships. Not rare many drug users end up engaging in risk and illicit activities, as prostitution and robbery, in an attempt to obtain resources to continue to use the drug [8–10].

Due to this cocaine consume aspects, as well as addiction and other problems from this condition, the cocaine dependence should be studied in a multicenter and multidisciplinary way involving diverse knowledge on areas such as chemistry, pharmacology, psychology, and social sciences. Cocaine chemical dependence is one of the most difficult pathologies to treat, and the discussion about this theme should be constantly emphasized.

2. Cocaine forms of presentation

Cocaine's purified form has a pearly white color. Being a weak alkaline compound, it can combine with acids forming many types of salts. Cocaine hydrochloride (COC) is the main common salt; besides, other types of salts can be found such as sulfate, nitrate, borate, and salicylate. Different salts dissolve in a high or low extension in different solvents. The COC salt is polar and highly soluble in water. However, molecular form of cocaine, popularly called free base, is the opposite of salt forms and is practically insoluble in water (**Figure 1**) [11, 12].

The terms "coca paste" or "crude coca paste" and "coca base" are similar in relation to the active principle presence; however, they differ in chemical waste products used in the extraction from coca leaves. While "coca paste" still has many waste products, "coca base" comes from withdrawal of such waste products. Nevertheless, these terms are used indistinctly by own coca farms and drug producers [3, 13, 14].

The coca base is smoked by the drug user and such use form began in Peru in the beginning of the 1970s and spread to other producers' countries, such as Colombia and Bolivia, during the same decade. After that, the drug use reached the other countries of South America, including border regions of Brazil with producer's countries. In the Andean countries, Coca base, when smoked isolatedly is called "basuco", and in Argentina, the drug is called "paco". When the drug is smoked with tobacco or marijuana, it is called "grimmie" [3, 15].

Merla is made by coca paste or coca base mixed with sodium carbonate (Na_2CO_3) and sulfuric acid (H_2SO_4), dissolved in a heated aqueous solution with kerosene. Merla is smoked usually mixed with tobacco or marijuana [16, 17].

Cocaine is more usually found as a crystalline powder, COC, obtained through coca base treatment with hydrochloric acid (HCl). In this form, it can be smoked, because it cannot be vaporized and decomposes with temperature increasing. Usually, cocaine is self-administrated by nasal aspiration or orally or intravenously [17]. The COC receives many popular denominations such as "powder," "snow,"

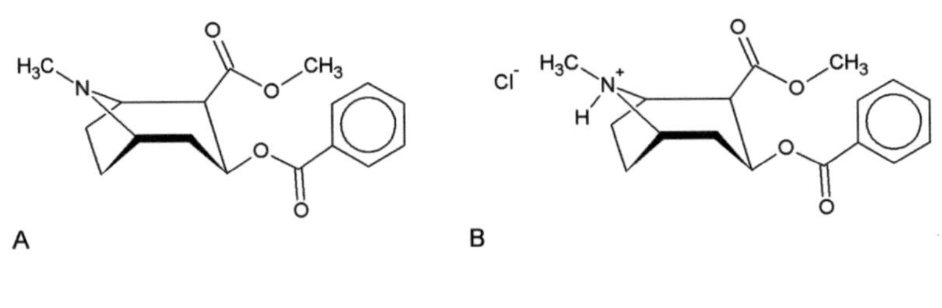

Figure 1.
Cocaine chemical structures in its molecular form (A) and its main salt form, cocaine hydrochloride (B).

"coke," "flour," etc. Besides, all these terms refer to the drug as a white powder, paved, and bright, which, after powdered with the help of a barber blade or a plastic card, can be snorted or diluted in water and injected intravenously with a syringe and needle [18]. The practice of injecting cocaine is commonly known as "peak" in Latin America countries [19].

Freebasing is a cocaine derivate product, which consists of COC converted to molecular form of cocaine. For this, COC is treated with an alkaline solution such as ammonia hydroxide (NH_4OH) or sodium bicarbonate ($NaHCO_3$) to remove HCl. This process needs a mixture of diethyl ether with water under heating. The material originated is crushed and smoked in improvised pipes. This cocaine form of presentation is usually made in a low scale for own use. Due to the use of diethyl ether in the process of heating, explosion accidents occurred, causing risk of life of the person who manufactured the drug, leading to disuse of this form of presentation [20].

Crack cocaine can be obtained from the freebasing with the removal of diethyl ether and adding NH_4OH or $NaHCO_3$ and water under moderate heating. Under these conditions, cocaine precipitates in an almost pure product after solvent evaporation. Crack cocaine obtainment process can be also from COC, coca paste, or coca base. From COC, the drug is diluted in hot water or in NH_4OH or $NaHCO_3$ solutions with posterior removal of diluent layer at the end of the process. From coca paste or coca base, the drug is heated with $NaHCO_3$ solution without removal of final diluents, resulting in low concentrated and more "dirt" drug [16, 21, 22]. The name "crack" comes from the crackling noise that the drug produces during heating. The drug is smoked in improvised pipes, tin cans, or plastic tubes. Crack cocaine also can be smoked mixed with marijuana (merged or "mesclado") or tobacco ("pitilho") [23, 24].

Oxi is a cocaine form of presentation obtained by coca paste treatment with lime (CaO) or cement, H_2SO_4, kerosene, gasoline, and other substances. The drug is smoked in improvised pipes or mixed with tobacco. The term "oxi" or "oxidized" originated due to the suspected use of oxidant agents as a way to remove impurities during initial process of drug fabrication. There seems to be a superposition between oxi and crack cocaine related to its use patterns; however, unfolding remains unknown [25].

"Virado" or "turned powder" consists in transforming crack cocaine rock into a powder adding boric acid (H_3BO_3). This mixture is heated to assist the process and subsequently cooled and made into powder, which is snorted similar to COC. The "virado" is cocaine in borate salt form, which is absorbed by the nasal mucosa [26].

Table 1 presents main cocaine forms of presentation related to its chemical forms and use forms, and **Figure 2** shows main consumed forms of presentation.

3. Pharmacological mechanisms

Absorption velocity and maximum plasma concentration are dependent on administration routes in which cocaine self-administration occurs. These routes can be oral, intravenous, intranasal (snorted), and respiratory (smoked), being the latter two most common [27, 28].

Cocaine smoked in its molecular form promotes faster absorption of the drug, through pulmonary absorption. This results in faster appearance and high intensity effects in the drug user, when compared with intravenous route. Kinetic patterns of both routes are similar. Usually, smoked route effects occur in 3–5 seconds, with maximum plasma concentration of 300–900 $ng \cdot mL^{-1}$. Maximum intensity of effects occurs in almost 3 minutes, lasting approximately 5–10 minutes. Observations of these phenomena are extremely important, since cocaine use in this route can lead to dependence in a very short period of drug use [29–31].

Popular name	Chemical form	Use form
Coca paste	Molecular	Smoked
Coca base	Molecular	Smoked
Basuco	Molecular	Smoked
Paco	Molecular	Smoked
Merla	Molecular	Smoked
Powder	Salt	Snorted or injected
Freebasing	Molecular	Smoked
Crack cocaine	Molecular	Smoked
Oxi	Molecular	Smoked
"Virado"	Salt	Snorted

Table 1.
Main cocaine forms of presentation and its chemical forms and use forms.

The efficiency of smoking act in relation to drug chemical availability in the body and in relation to the speed and quantity of cocaine in the bloodstream in conditions to produce the desired effect depends on a number of factors, such as amount of drug burned, temperature used for burning, the container used for heating, and condensing of the drug in containers used for smoking. Absorption rate is high because extensive superficial area of the lungs is highly vascularized. When cocaine is smoked, the formation of the anhydroecgonine methyl ester (AEME) occurs, a cocaine thermal degradation by-product, which is eliminated in the urine and can be used as a chemical marker of this form of use [32, 33].

Intranasal administration also called "snort" or "cafungar" consists in arranging cocaine salt lined up on smooth surface, each row with approximately 10–30 mg, which is aspirated in such a way that absorption occurs through the nasal mucosa. Cocaine use by this route or by the oral mucosa propitiates absorption through the nasopharyngeal membranes, with low absorption rate due to the vasoconstrictor drug properties. The administration by this route produces smaller plasma levels for a longer time due to slow absorption rate. Approximately 20–30% of the administered drug is absorbed. Maximum plasma concentration occurs, on average, 30 minutes after drug administration and is conditioned by differences in technical effectiveness of aspiration and partial dose swallowing; besides individual characteristics of each user, this produces different levels of mucosal vasoconstriction and possibility of biotransformation in the mucosa itself [17]. Although effects appear slowly, the magnitude is comparable to the intravenous route. Doses of approximately 0.4 $mg \cdot kg^{-1}$ of body weight (30–40 mg) are associated with a maximum plasma concentration of 50 $ng \cdot mL^{-1}$, while those corresponding to 1–2 $mg \cdot kg^{-1}$ are associated to 100–200 $ng \cdot mL^{-1}$ [29, 30].

The oral route is also effective in terms of drug chemical stability and bioavailability. After approximately 30 minutes, when there is no plasma detection, gastrointestinal absorption quickly occurs and maximum plasma concentration usually occurs between 45 and 90 minutes. Delay in oral absorption, in relation to what occurs in intranasal route, is due to ionization of cocaine in the stomach acidic environment, and the delay in reaching the small intestine basic medium, region where the molecular form prevails, leads to a higher absorption rate [34–36].

Injectable cocaine has its beginning of action about 30–45 seconds after administration. The "peak," as this form of use is known, produces an effect called rush

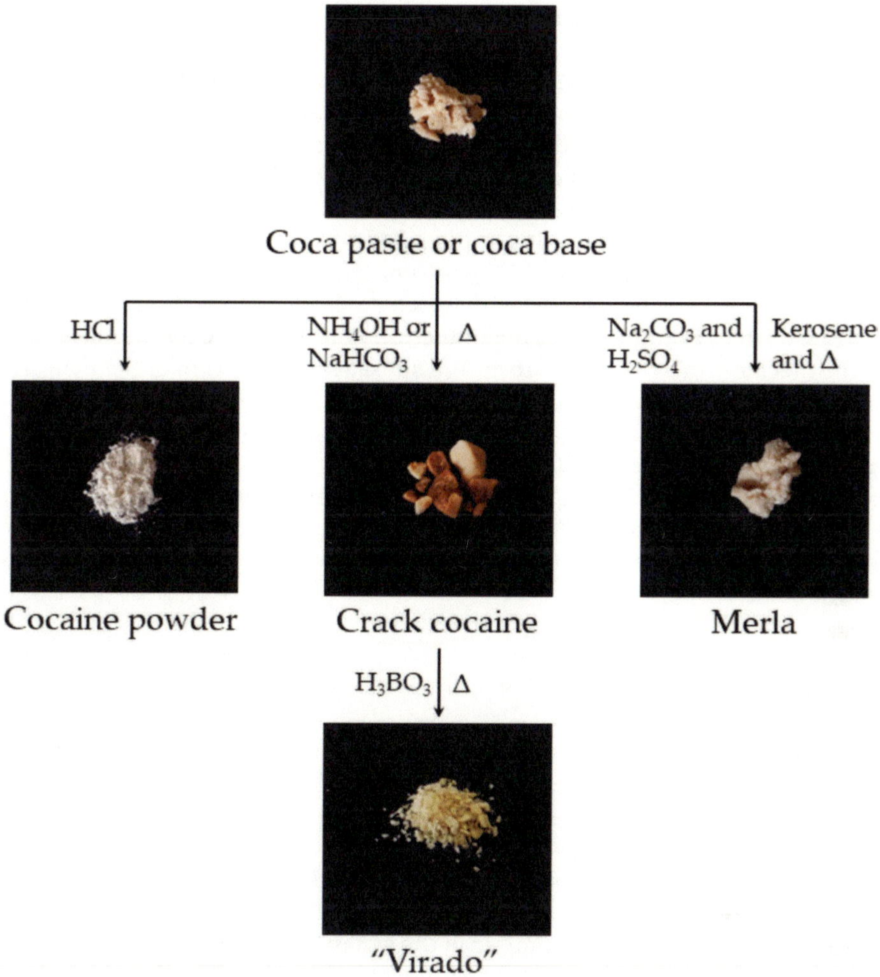

Figure 2.
Cocaine most consumed forms of presentation. HCl = hydrochloric acid; NH_4OH = ammonium hydroxide; $NaHCO_3$ = sodium bicarbonate; Na_2CO_3 = sodium carbonate; H_2SO_4 = sulfuric acid; H_3BO_3 = boric acid; Δ = heating.

or "baque" [12]. To be injected cocaine is usually diluted in water and heated to facilitate dissolution or filtered on cotton to avoid impurities. This route does not pass through the absorption stage and through the hepatic first pass effect. Thus, the cocaine available in bloodstream is almost 100%, requiring a dose 20% lower than that ingested or snorted. Duration of effects is about 20 minutes [37, 38].

Bioavailability of smoked cocaine is approximately 70% due to losses of 30% of thermal decomposition or condensation in the utensil used for this purpose [15]. Intranasal bioavailability is reported to be in the range of 60–80%. Although there is a delay in absorption by this route, the loss is relatively lower [37].

Because cocaine is a lipophilic substance, it can easily cross the blood-brain barrier (BBB), and experimental data suggest that the drug is caught by adipocytes and consequently accumulates in the central nervous system (CNS) [39]. There are placental transfer and milk secretion. Placental transfer has passive transport characteristics due to drug lipophilic properties [40]. Cocaine presence may also occur in the drug user's semen regardless of administration route used [41].

Kinetic parameters and plasma half-life of elimination (T½) for cocaine vary according to the administration route. For the snorted route, T½ is around

50–78 minutes; for the smoked route, it is around 38–58 minutes, and for intravenous route, it is around 40–67 minutes [20, 34, 37].

Cocaine recreational doses lead to temporary elevations in noradrenaline (NA) and dopamine (DA) concentrations with subsequent reduction to below normal values. These variations in these neurotransmitter concentrations are related, respectively, to states of euphoria and depression experienced by the drug users [28, 30].

The main mechanism of action of cocaine in the CNS is blocking the reuptake of DA in synaptic clefts, due to cocaine binding to dopamine transporter sites. Dopamine accumulation at D1 and D2 postsynaptic receptors seems to be the pathophysiological mechanism through which euphoria occurs. The consequence of neurotransmitter accumulation is the induction of presynaptic receptors, resulting from the mechanism of self-regulation and subsequent depletion of the neurotransmitter. Similarly, adrenergic stimulation seems to occur by the same mechanism, and as a result of chronic use of cocaine, both NA and DA become significantly reduced in the brain. Decreased DA in the brain may result in abnormalities of dopaminergic pathways, leading to psychiatric complications such as depression and bipolar disorder [42–44]. The D2 receptor is present in higher concentration in the striatum and nucleus accumbens, and its stimulation has been associated with psychotic behavior [45–47].

4. Cocaine effects

There are several expected effects for the person who is using cocaine. Most common effects are loss of appetite, increased blood pressure, nausea, anxiety, and/or paranoia. It is important to remember that such effects are in accordance with the singularity of the person.

Cocaine psychoactive effects arise from increased neuronal activity of DA and NA, stimulating brain reward pathway. Blocking of dopamine reuptake increases concentration of this neurotransmitter in the synaptic cleft, producing a more intense pleasure sensation [48, 49]. The intensity of pleasure is so high that the sensations are difficult to describe [50].

Psychic effects caused by cocaine use occur in two distinct ways and always manifest in the same sequence. Initially, cocaine positive effects, in other words, pleasure sensations, occur due to concentration increase of DA and NA. Such sensations are replaced by negative effects or unpleasant sensations, like paranoia, due to DA and NA depletion. Positive effects emerge more quickly, decreasing their intensity until the appearance of negative effects [49–51].

Paranoia is a constant sensation due to cocaine use, especially in its smoked form, crack cocaine. Paranoia is responsible for most of conflicts witnessed among crack cocaine users. This paranoia is a consequence of the intense use in which the inhalation of large amounts induces irritability feelings, tremors, and bizarre attitudes [52]. It manifests as a constant restlessness, usually accompanied by a sense of fear in drug users, who start to watch the place where they are using the drug, showing great distrust of each other and in relation to the people who are nearby [53].

In an ethnographic study, held in the city of São Paulo—Brazil, the sense of "radiation" for the research participants was described. The "radiation" means discord, mistrust, fear, in the scene of crack cocaine use. It is the breaking of reciprocity, thief, betrayal, trust abuse, and disrespect [54].

Combination of pharmacological and sociocultural effects identified in crack cocaine use determines the risk that these drug users can undergo. Crack cocaine causes a state of ecstasy of short duration, being one of the main characteristics for its risk of addiction. Constant consumption becomes compulsive, and the need to acquire the drug takes on a more important place than family, job, social relationship, self-care, etc. This relationship of potent and short duration effects, together with permanent need to acquire money to obtain the drug, combined with the illegality of this practice (and its consequences of further exclusion of users), articulate to the prevalence of compulsive use among crack cocaine users [55].

This ability of crack cocaine to develop an almost instantaneous addiction framework has always been pointed out as unquestionable truth. Although this information is widely disseminated, it has never been scientifically tested. It was identified that, when compared to the numbers on abusive use of COC, crack cocaine users have a higher percentage of recurrence in use. This relationship may be associated to the fact that crack cocaine is more accessible in poor communities, where COC is economically less viable [48]. **Table 2** shows main health problems that cocaine users can develop in the short and long term.

5. Forms of cocaine use

Over the years, there has been an increase in the variety of forms of presentation and consumption of cocaine. By identifying a psychoactive substance, different ways are discovered to achieve the desired effects, making it one more market product in our society. In recent decades, cocaine use in its different forms of presentation has taken on worrying dimensions, with serious consequences for the users, their families, and communities, wrecking different interfaces of daily life [56–58]. Cocaine consumption represents a constant search for novelty, main characteristic of the current society of consumption [24].

Understanding the ways of how people use cocaine, materials used, as well as different ways of using this substance are of fundamental importance to identify contexts of greater or lesser vulnerability to drug consumption.

It is difficult to find cocaine use isolated. Usually, the drug is consumed in conjunction with others. In the state of São Paulo—Southeast of Brazil, there is a greater prevalence of crack cocaine use associated with alcohol and/or marijuana. These associations appear as a strategy to minimize risks caused by crack cocaine compulsive use. This is because alcohol or marijuana alleviates crack cocaine craving symptoms [59, 60]. In the state of Pernambuco—Northeast of Brazil, this

Short-term effects	Long-term effects
Loss of appetite	Cognitive problems
Increase in blood pressure	Sexual dysfunction
Nausea	Renal and pulmonary damage
Anxiety and paranoia	Nasal septum destruction
Depression	Tooth wear
Dilated pupils	Disorientation and apathy
Disturbed sleep	Brain hemorrhage
Erratic behavior	Irregular heartbeat
Euphoria	
Auditory and tactile hallucinations	
Tremors	

Table 2.
Main health problems that can be developed by cocaine users.

consumption pattern was also identified; however, the use of the "shot," only crack cocaine smoked isolated, still appears as a preference for most drug users [61].

"Virado" or turned powder is a cocaine-differentiated use form in the culture of cocaine use in Brazil, especially in the state of Pernambuco. Some studies pointed this form of use as characteristic of Pernambuco [26, 62, 63], not being registered, yet, in any other state of Brazil or another country [61].

"Virado" consumption has more a social characterization, being used mainly in festive and celebration environments, not stigmatizing so much people who consume this form of presentation. "Virado" has a longer effect, similar to COC snorted, not causing so much compulsivity as crack cocaine smoked. Despite these positive aspects, "virado" causes significant nasal bleeding, and for sharing objects for aspiration, such as plastic straw, this increases infectious disease contamination probability, such as DST/AIDS [61].

Not recognizing possibility of other forms of cocaine use is denying entire social and cultural process involved in drug use issues. Adaptations of the drug users are strategies built from social exchanges that occur at the time of use. New forms of use do not arise in an isolated way, not depending only on the effects of cocaine and or on individual's collective constructions. They are fruits of social dynamics established between the groups, which can make viable different forms of use more or less harmful [24].

6. Psychosocial treatment

There are several types of therapeutic approaches that can be used to treat people with cocaine use problems. Complex conditions of drug use contexts, social and personal implications associated with the use, and users' biopsychosocial conditions have required tools and care strategies. This allows a varied therapeutic offer, which aims to reach people with this problem in an integrated way. Thus, treatment must be prepared to offer a myriad of interventions to the multiple needs showed, through personalized and singular indications. Application of associated and multidisciplinary approaches presents better therapeutic results [64, 65]. We will focus on psychosocial treatments, and the following will present some approaches of psychosocial treatments indicated for cocaine addiction.

6.1 Cognitive behavioral therapy

Cognitive behavioral therapy (CBT) has been shown to be an effective approach in chemical dependence treatment. CBT is defined as a set of semistructured interventions, objective and goal-oriented. It is based on the assumption that cognitions, emotions, and thoughts are among the factors considered as precipitators or maintainers of behavior. Thus, several techniques and protocols are used, addressing central themes that involve relation of the person with the drug and specific themes to each person. It is fundamental that the professional is well trained for the model application, planning activities according to needs of each person [64]. CBT supports dependent people to become abstinent or reducing drug use, allowing them to recognize risk situations, to avoid them, and to deal with problems associated with cocaine use [66]. From this approach, other variations that explore motivational and behavioral aspects were derived.

6.1.1 Motivational interview

Motivational interview (MI) consists of a counseling approach used to promote behavior change, according to individual interests of lifestyle enhancement. This approach adds value at every stage of treatment and can be associated with other techniques. It is based on concepts of motivation, ambivalence, and readiness for change. Such concepts imply in the presence of three professional attitudes: collaboration, evocation and respect for the autonomy [64]. MI interventions are more persuasive than coercive; more empathetic and welcoming than confrontational. In this perspective, relapse is perceived as a key event for motivational process, generating self-efficacy increase [67].

6.1.2 Relapse prevention

In relapse prevention (RP) model, addictive behaviors are bad habits that can be changed. These people are considered to have learned these behaviors and thoughts that are dysfunctional, and even though problems are generated for them, drugs are still used when the user has to deal with difficult situations. It is assumed that the person did not develop or learned more adaptive behaviors that generate gratification or enable them to solve problems differently. RP is based on three fundamental points: (i) awareness of the problem, (ii) facing skills training, and (iii) lifestyle modification [68, 69]. In RP, all aspects involved in the relapse process are considered. Thus, the person has the opportunity to subjects such as facing strategies aiming at training their self-efficacy to develop skills for handling similar situations in the future [64].

6.1.3 Social skills training

It is presented as a set of interventions, which aims to develop and improve cognitive and behavioral skills to change drug use behavior. Social skills are a set of behaviors expressed by a person in self-social environment, which include expressing feelings, desires, attitudes, opinions, or rights, appropriate to situation, adaptively and assertively, decreasing the probability of future difficulties arising. These skills should be understood in their social context, variations in communication pattern, specific situations, age, sex, social class, education, and purpose. Social skills training and drug use show that these people have deficits in such behaviors, which can be considered an important risk factor for drug use, highlighting the possibility of lack of assertiveness and communication strategies for drug resistance and negotiation. Thus, it is understood that the drug becomes a mean of facing external pressures, everyday events, and interpersonal situations, without need to express assertive behavior. Obtaining a good repertoire of socially skillful behaviors is related to lower risk of drug use [70].

6.1.4 Contingency management

This treatment aims to promote abstinence and other desired behaviors by organizing systematic rewards in alternative behavior occurrence incompatible with drug use. It is based on the theory of operant conditioning. Contingency management (CM) has been a key technique in solving problems by inhibiting responses. In the therapeutic relationship, the therapist has the possibility of reinforcing or punishing patient's advancement or problem behaviors. Thus, CM is a behavioral treatment aimed to change individual repertoire and decrease or extinguish undesirable behaviors. It can be used associated with other therapeutic approaches [64, 66].

6.2 Psychosocial approaches

For treatment of people who have problems in cocaine abuse, it can be seen that problems themselves are highly particular needs. Thus, the health professional must demonstrate skills and availability. There is a need for treatment spaces that stimulate creativity, freedom, and autonomy to the team for mental health work of cocaine users, as well as practices constitution that allow the user to be the focus of therapy in detriment to substance use. Therefore, it is necessary to establish solid therapeutic links; this is recognized by establishment of a solidary and trusting relationship, so that the health professional understands host as an important strategy for care development [71]. These multiprofessional services care, with extended models called psychosocial, in addition to continued care, may increase chances of adherence and positive response in terms of behavior change. This is the expanded clinic proposes that the person should be well received and addressed their unique needs, through shared construction of the singular therapeutic project [72].

6.3 Mindfulness

Conventional treatment, when combined with different approaches such as, acupuncture and image replacement techniques, physical exercise and cooperative games, promotes decreased anxiety; craving relief; relapse prevention; integration, socialization and obtaining another form of pleasure, in case of physical exercise and cooperative games [73]. Relationship between stress and dependence is well known. Stress increases probability of using alcohol and other drugs and may precipitate relapses. It is necessary to incorporate techniques of stress control in patients in outpatient treatment [74, 75]. Mindfulness has been described as a practice of learning to focus attention on momentary experience an attitude of curiosity, openness, and acceptance. Mindfulness practices have become increasingly popular in complementary therapeutic strategies for a variety of medical and psychiatric conditions [76].

6.4 Harm reduction

Harm reduction (HR) actions constitute a set of public health measures aimed at minimizing adverse consequences of drug use. The fundamental principle guiding HR is respect for freedom of choice, as studies and experience in health services show that many drug users, sometimes, cannot or do not want to stop using drugs and, even so, they need that risks from drug use to be minimized. HR is still perceived as a strategy to guarantee the rights of people who use drugs, regardless of whether or not to stop using [77].

More than just an approach, HR is presented as an ethical policy of respect for integrality, autonomy, and human rights. In this sense, it becomes a professional stance that permeates all activities, hosting, and services organization, including through guidance and contact with families in domiciliary visits and activities carried out in primary health care. For HR, the drug is not the determining agent for care construction, so that evidences are considered that relation of the person with the drug does not necessarily always occur in a relation of dependence. Instead, various possibilities of relation of the person with the drug are thought that extend objectives of its practices. Thus, it was highlighted that even though HR is currently linked to the world of drugs, it is a way of acting and of caring present in human relations [78].

7. Drug user recursion

Even with psychosocial treatments available for cocaine addiction described above, it is observed that, although they reduce severity of psychosocial problems caused to cocaine users, these models failed to respond to the phenomenon of "relapse." The model of "prevention of relapse" is only operationalized by biomedical bias, awaiting positive and unique outcome of total abstinence of drug use. Such model of care and attention ends up being insufficient in face of other proposals of care that do not operate in the same perspective. This is the case of models such as HR based on human rights, social constructionism, and psychosocial treatment itself that accept other possibilities of outcome of cases as, for example, controlled drug use.

Thus, the "recursion" is presented as an alternative of reflection and more consistent policy action with these other models and perspectives of care. In the case to the phenomenon of "relapse" another reflexive paradigm emerges: recursion as a principle and theoretical construct of Morin's Theory of Complexity [79–81] and reflected in a practical way by Maturana [82–84].

Consequently, "recursion" can be understood as repetition that occurs in all processes and living systems [80, 82, 83]. A permanent and endless movement, in people, occurs from their personal experiences, with their own senses and meanings to each one who lives their own recursive movement [85]. These experiments are based on explanations that each person can print to their personal movement [82, 83]. Such explanations try to "justify" or "enlight" the drug users about what they had been going through in their lives.

Therefore, the idea of "recursion" as a new challenge to understanding the phenomenon of "relapse" considers characteristic aspects of the person and circumstances of his narratives in continuing resignifications, during and after the "relapse" process.

To better understand the "recursion" as a "reupdating" motion constant in the life history of people who use drugs, which go beyond "return to a substance use pattern," we cite the work of Cruz et al. [86] that say: "Now, in relation to the principle of recursion, this is explicit among people who use drugs, in which one perceives abstinence moments interspersed with a pattern of intense consumption of the drug. So, the notion of recursion refers to movement of traversing again, having, many times, an inexhaustible back-and-forth movement of actions and implementations. The principle of recursion is a process in which effects are at same time causers and producers of the process itself".

Starting from complexity theory, besides the principle of "recursion," we find others that are important to understand the behavior of drug users. We also highlight the principle of systems theory. This is directly related to functioning of people and their families. Systems theory is widely used to understand functioning of various social systems, in particular those of family relations, for studying feedback mechanisms between self-regulating systems [87].

In systems theory, fundamental attributes of the organism are parts of the whole. And the whole will always be greater than its parts—a reflection also used by Gestalt Therapy [88]. Thus, one sees the organized assembly of parts that form a complex and dynamic whole, concluding that every system is a subsystem of a larger system. And since a system is larger than the sum of the parts, its influence is incessant with environment, so that it not only maintains its organization but also modifies it, seeking change and not just opposing it [87].

It is perceived the principle of recursion, as part of a new paradigm that acts with argument of active organization and constant reorganization [79]. For Rameh-de Albuquerque [85], the preceding "re" implies articulation of linked knowledge: "[...] repeat, reflect, revolve, rearrange, reproduce, return, recall, repeat... Relapse?! What is recurrent in think? That when the drug user relapses, he returns to the same place from which he left. However, in the light of recursion, he no longer returns to the same point. Your passage through experience represents somehow a new learning."

Hence, the difference between the "relapse" construct and the idea of "recursion" is the fact that in "recursion" we do not expect a definitive outcome due the multiple process repetion possibilities each person experiences. When passing through a drug use experience, the person remeans what happens to him and can, on the other hand, produce new learning that will encourage him to have a new relationship with the use of drugs.

Thus, considering reflections of Maturana and Varela [89] that all coupling and interaction directly affect the nervous system due to the structural changes that arouse in it, we consider that all experience is transformative, even so, sometimes, changes are not completely visible. Such reflections make even greater sense in relation to humans, and we can transpose this idea to expand our understanding of the phenomenon of "relapse."

Every "relapse" brings learning that we cannot always see. And considering the biomedical perspective of care, which seeks abstinence as the only possibility of successful treatment outcome, the idea of considering other learning and ways of dealing with drug use is not accepted. Generally, the treatments offered are anchored in other paradigms as already mentioned above. In the abstinence paradigm, "partial" learning of the person who uses drugs is not accepted. The resignification that is given by each person is not accepted. Do not consider his experience with the drug and use contexts involved. That way, the proposal to consider "recursion" as something inherent in all living systems, regardless of drug use or abuse, strengthens and connects with the perspective of other treatment models.

HR, for example, will accept "partial" learning considering possibility of restructuring the subject from a more controlled use and less harmful to your health and to the social and family relations, facilitating adherence of many people who do not want or cannot stop using drugs [90].

8. Conclusions

Cocaine has several forms of presentation. These modifications in forms of presentation can cause changes in the molecule of cocaine, which generates different drug kinetic and dynamic patterns. Cocaine in its salt form is usually administered snorted and has less intense and longer effects. In its molecular form, usually smoked, effects are more intense and short. These variations in intensity and duration of effects end up influencing use frequency and onset of addiction.

Cocaine addiction is a rather difficult pathology to treat, and there are several approaches such as medication, religious, and psychosocial treatment. There are psychosocial approaches that derive from cognitive behavioral therapy, in addition to other approaches that consider individual rights as harm reduction. Nevertheless, these approaches do not study the phenomenon of relapse. Recursion comprises the phenomenon of relapse as something natural in the process of treatment of the drug user and as a form of learning, being these elements essential for the addiction treatment.

The phenomenon of cocaine addiction is complex and involves from chemical and pharmacological characteristics of the substance to its contexts of use. New understandings of various forms of drug presentation in the world and new treatment models need to be constantly discussed.

Conflict of interest

The authors report no conflicts of interest. The authors alone are responsible for the content and writing of this chapter.

Author details

Antonio Gomes de Castro Neto[1*], Magda da Silva Figueiroa[2],
Renata Barreto Fernandes de Almeida[3], Rossana Carla Rameh-de-Albuquerque[4],
Iandê dos Santos Gomes de Moura[5] and Solange Aparecida Nappo[6]

1 Federal University of Pernambuco, Recife, Brazil

2 City Hall of the City of Recife, Recife, Brazil

3 University Center UniFavip/Wyden, Caruaru, Brazil

4 Federal Institute of Pernambuco, Recife, Brazil

5 Catholic University of Pernambuco, Recife, Brazil

6 Federal University of São Paulo, São Paulo, Brazil

*Address all correspondence to: litaree@yahoo.com

References

[1] United Nations Office on Drugs and Crime. World Drug Report 2017—Market Analysis of Plant-Based Drugs: Opiates, Cocaine, Cannabis. Vienna: United Nations Publication; 2017. 68 p. ISBN: 978-92-1-148291-1, eISBN: 978-92-1-060623-3

[2] Acock MC, Lyndon J, Johnson E, Collins R. Effects of temperature and light levels on leaf yield and cocaine content in two *Erythroxylum* species. Annals of Botany. 1996;**78**:49-53. DOI: 10.1006/anbo.1996.0094

[3] Casale JF, Klein RF. Illicit production of cocaine. Forensic Science Review. 1993;**5**:95-107

[4] United Nations Office on Drugs and Crime. World Drug Report 2010. Vienna: United Nations publication; 2010. 313 p. ISBN: 978-92-1-148256-0

[5] Nestler E. The neurobiology of cocaine addiction. Science & Practice Perspectives. 2005;**3**:4-10

[6] Hummel M, Unterwald EM. D1 dopamine receptor: A putative neurochemical and behavioral link to cocaine action. Journal of Cellular Physiology. 2002;**191**:17-27. DOI: 10.1002/jcp.10078

[7] Nutt D, King LA, Saulsbury W, Blakemore C. Development of a rational scale to assess the harm of drugs of potential misuse. Lancet. 2007;**369**:1047-1053. DOI: 10.1016/S0140-6736(07)60464-4

[8] Duailibi LB, Ribeiro M, Laranjeira R. Profile of cocaine and crack users in Brazil. Cadernos de Saúde Pública. 2008;**24**:S545-S557. DOI: 10.1590/S0102-311X2008001600007

[9] Wang L, Min JE, Krebs E, Evans E, Huang D, Liu L, et al. Polydrug use and its association with drug treatment outcomes among primary heroin, methamphetamine, and cocaine users. The International Journal on Drug Policy;**201749**:32-40. DOI: 10.1016/j.drugpo.2017.07.009

[10] Bisch NK, Moreira TC, Benchaya MC, Pozza DR, Freitas LCN, Farias MS, et al. Telephone counseling for young Brazilian cocaine and/or crack users. Who are these users? Jornal de Pediatria. 2011;**32**:31-39. DOI: 10.1016/j.jped.2017.12.016

[11] Singh S. Chemistry, design, and structure—Activity relationship of cocaine antagonists. Chemical Reviews. 2000;**100**:925-1024. DOI: 10.1021/cr9700538

[12] Pharmacology Education Partnership. Acids, Bases and Cocaine Addicts [Internet]. 2016. Available from: https://sites.duke.edu/thepepproject/files/2016/01/PEP_M1.pdf [Accessed: June 25, 2018]

[13] Pascale A, Negrin A, Laborde A. Pasta base de cocaína: Experiencia del Centro de Información y Asesoramiento Toxicológico. Adicciones. 2010;**22**:227-232. DOI: 10.20882/adicciones.183

[14] López-Hill X, Prieto JP, Meikle MN, Urbanavicius J, Abin-Carriquiry JA, Prunell G, et al. Coca-paste seized samples characterization: Chemical analysis, stimulating effect in rats and relevance of caffeine as a major adulterant. Behavioural Brain Research. 2011;**221**: 134-141. DOI: 10.1016/j.bbr.2011.03.005

[15] Pascale A, Hynes M, Cumsille F, Bares C. Use of Cocaine Base Paste in South America: A Review of Epidemiological, Medical and Toxicological Issues. Organization of American States/Inter-American Drug Abuse Control Commission: Washington; 2014. 28 p. ISBN: 978-0-8270-6165-1

[16] Blickman T. Smokeable Cocaine and Crack in Brazil—A Quick Scan of the Market [Internet]. 2006. Available from: https://www.tni.org/files/crack-brazil.pdf [Accessed: June 25, 2018]

[17] Gootenberg P. Cocaine powder and crack cocaine—A changeable history? In: Brownstein HH, editor. The Handbook of Drugs and Society. Chichester: Wiley; 2015. p. 90-108. DOI:10.1002/9781118726761

[18] Drug Enforcement Administration. Cocaine (Street Names: Coke, Snow, Crack, Rock) [Internet]. 2013. Available from: http://www.deadiversiontest.usdoj.gov/drug_chem_info/cocaine.pdf [Accessed: June 25, 2018]

[19] Sanchez ZM, Nappo SA. Progression on drug use and its intervening factors among crack users. Revista de Saúde Pública. 2002;**36**:420-430. DOI: 10.1590/S0034-89102002000400007

[20] Freebase Cocaine FE. High bioavailability with increase in potency. In: Freye E, Levy JV, editors. Pharmacology and Abuse of Cocaine, Amphetamines, Ecstasy and Related Designer Drugs. Dordrecht: Springer; 2009. pp. 43-47. DOI: 10.1007/978-90-481-2448-0_7

[21] Cornish JW, O'Brien CP. Crack cocaine abuse: An epidemic with many public health consequences. Annual Review of Public Health. 1996;**17**:259-273

[22] Butler AJ, Rehm J, Fischer B. Health outcomes associated with crack-cocaine use: Systematic review and meta-analyses. Drug and Alcohol Dependence. 2017;**180**:401-416. DOI: 10.1016/j.drugalcdep.2017.08.036

[23] Dias AC, Araújo MR, Laranjeira R. Evolution of drug use in a cohort of treated crack cocaine users. Revista de Saúde Pública. 2011;**45**:938-948. DOI: 10.1590/S0034-89102011005000049

[24] Jorge MSB, Quinderé PHD, Yasui S, Albuquerque RA. The ritual of crack consumption: Socio-anthropological aspects and impacts on the health of users. Ciência & Saúde Coletiva. 2013;**18**:2909-2918. DOI: 10.1590/S1413-81232013001000015

[25] Silva-Junior RC, Gomes CS, Goulart-Júnior SS, Almeida FV, Grobério TS, Braga JWB, et al. Demystifying "oxi" cocaine: Chemical profiling analysis of a "new Brazilian drug" from Acre state. Forensic Science International. 2012;**221**:113-119. DOI: 10.1016/j.forsciint.2012.04.015

[26] Nappo SA, Sanchez ZM, Rameh R, Almeida R, Uchôa R. Virado: A new method of crack consumption in Brazil. The American Journal on Addictions. 2012;**21**(6):1-2. DOI: 10.1111/j.1521-0391.2012.00272.x

[27] Barnett G, Hawks R, Resnick R. Cocaine pharmacokinetics in humans. Journal of Ethnopharmacology. 1981;**3**:353-366. DOI: 10.1016/0378-8741(81)90063-5

[28] Freye E. Pharmacology of cocaine. In: Freye E, Levy JV, editors. Pharmacology and Abuse of Cocaine, Amphetamines, Ecstasy and Related Designer Drugs. Dordrecht: Springer; 2009. pp. 49-60. DOI: 10.1007/978-90-481-2448-0_7

[29] Javaid JI, Fischman MW, Schuster CR, Dekirmenjian H, Davis JM. Cocaine plasma concentration: Relation to physiological and subjective effects in humans. Science. 1978;**202**:227-228

[30] Ellefsen K, Concheiro M, Pirard S, Gorelick DA, Huestis MA. Pharmacodynamic effects and relationships to plasma and oral fluid pharmacokinetics after intravenous cocaine administration. Drug and Alcohol Dependence. 2016;**163**:116-125. DOI: 10.1016/j.drugalcdep.2016.04.004

[31] Fiorentin TR, D'Avila FB, Comiran E, Zamboni A, Scherer JN, Pechansky F, et al. Simultaneous determination of cocaine/crack and its metabolites in oral fluid, urine and plasma by liquid chromatography-mass spectrometry and its application in drug users. Journal of Pharmacological and Toxicological Methods. 2017;**86**:60-66. DOI: 10.1016/j.vascn.2017.04.003

[32] Garcia RCT, Torres LH, Balestrin NT, Andrioli TC, Flório JC, Oliveira CDR, et al. Anhydroecgonine methyl ester, a cocaine pyrolysis product, may contribute to cocaine behavioral sensitization. Toxicology. 2017;**376**: 44-50. DOI: 10.1016/j.tox.2016.04.009

[33] Takitane J, Leyton V, Andreuccetti G, Gjerde H, Vindenes V, Berg T. Determination of cocaine, metabolites and a crack cocaine biomarker in whole blood by liquid–liquid extraction and UHPLC–MS/MS. Forensic Science International. 2018;**289**:165-174. DOI: 10.1016/j.forsciint.2018.05.030

[34] Ma F, Falk JL, Lau CE. Cocaine pharmacodynamics after intravenous and oral administration in rats: Relation to pharmacokinetics. Psychopharmacology. 1999;**144**:323-332

[35] Lau CE, Sun L, Wang Q, Simpao A, Falk JL. Oral cocaine pharmacokinetics and pharmacodynamics in a cumulative-dose regimen: Pharmacokinetic-pharmacodynamic modeling of concurrent operant and spontaneous behavior within an operant context. The Journal of Pharmacology and Experimental Therapeutics. 2000;**295**:634-643

[36] Walsh SL, Stoops WW, Moody DE, Lin SN, Bigelow GE. Repeated dosing with oral cocaine in humans: Assessment of direct effects, withdrawal and pharmacokinetics. Experimental and Clinical Psychopharmacology. 2009;**17**:205-216. DOI: 10.1037/a0016469

[37] Javaid JI, Musa MN, Fischman M, Schuster CR, Davis JM. Kinetics of cocaine in humans after intravenous and intranasal administration. Biopharmaceutics & Drug Disposition. 1983;**4**:9-18. DOI: 10.1002/bdd.2510040104

[38] Samaha AN, Li Y, Robinson TE. The rate of intravenous cocaine administration determines susceptibility to sensitization. The Journal of Neuroscience. 2002;**22**:3244-3250. DOI: 10.1523/JNEUROSCI.22-08-03244.2002

[39] Kousik SM, Napier TC, Carvey PM. The effects of psychostimulant drugs on blood brain barrier function and neuroinflammation. Frontiers in Pharmacology. 2012;**3**:1-12. DOI: 10.3389/fphar.2012.00121

[40] De Giovanni N, Marchetti D. Cocaine and its metabolites in the placenta: A systematic review of the literature. Reproductive Toxicology. 2012;**33**:1-14. DOI: 10.1016/j.reprotox.2011.10.012

[41] Cone EJ, Kato K, Hillsgrove M. Cocaine excretion in the semen of drug users. Journal of Analytical Toxicology. 1996;**20**:139-140

[42] Frank RA, Manderscheid PZ, Panicker S, Williams HP, Kokoris D. Cocaine euphoria, dysphoria, and tolerance assessed using drug-induced changes in brain-stimulation reward. Pharmacology, Biochemistry, and Behavior. 1992;**42**:771-779. DOI: 10.1016/0091-3057(92)90028-E

[43] Schank JR, Liles LC, Weinshenker D. Norepinephrine signaling through β-adrenergic receptors is critical for expression of cocaine-induced anxiety. Biological Psychiatry. 2008;**63**:1007-1012. DOI: 10.1016/j.biopsych.2007.10.018

[44] Ostlund SB, Halbout B. Mesolimbic dopamine signaling in cocaine

addiction. In: Preedy VR, editor. The Neuroscience of Cocaine—Mechanisms and Treatment. Cambridge: Academic Press; 2017. pp. 287-295. DOI: 10.1016/B978-0-12-803750-8.00029-4

[45] Dobbs LK, Kaplan AR, Lemos JC, Matsui A, Rubinstein M, Alvarez VA. Dopamine regulation of lateral inhibition between striatal neurons gates the stimulant actions of cocaine. Neuron. 2016;**90**:1100-1113. DOI: 10.1016/j.neuron.2016.04.031

[46] Perreault ML, Hasbi A, Shen MYF, Fan T, Navarro G, Flatcher PJ, et al. Disruption of a dopamine receptor complex amplifies the actions of cocaine. European Neuropsychopharmacology. 2016;**26**:1366-1377. DOI: 10.1016/j.euroneuro.2016.07.008

[47] Chen R, McIntosh S, Hemby SE, Sun H, Sexton T, Martin TJ, et al. High and low doses of cocaine intake are differentially regulated by dopamine D2 receptors in the ventral tegmental area and the nucleus accumbens. Neuroscience Letters. 2018;**671**:133-139. DOI: 10.1016/j.neulet.2018.02.026

[48] Morgan JP, Zimmer L. Social pharmacology of smokeable cocaine: Not all it's cracked up to be. In: Reinarman C, Levine HG, editors. Crack in America: Demon Drugs and Social Justice. London: University of California Press; 1997. pp. 131-170. ISBN: 0-520-20241-4

[49] Carlini EA, Nappo SA, Galduróz JCF, Noto AR. Drogas psicotrópicas—O que são e como agem. Revista IMESC. 2001;**3**:9-35

[50] Oliveira LG. Avaliação da cultura do uso de crack após uma década de introdução da droga na cidade de São Paulo [thesis]. São Paulo: Federal University of São Paulo; 2007

[51] Lacerda RB, Cruz MS, Nappo AS. Drogas estimulantes (anfetaminas, cocaína e outros): Efeitos agudos e crônicos. In: Formigoni MLOS, editor. Efeitos de substâncias psicoativas: Módulo 2. Brasília: Secretaria Nacional de Políticas sobre Drogas; 2016. pp. 1-144. ISBN: 978-85-85820-62-6

[52] Raupp LM. Circuitos de uso de crack nas cidades de São Paulo e Porto Alegre: Cotidiano, práticas e cuidado [thesis]. São Paulo: University of São Paulo; 2011

[53] Raupp LM, Adorno RCF. Circuitos de uso de crack na região central da cidade de São Paulo (SP, Brasil). Ciência & Saúde Coletiva. 2011;**16**:2613-2622. DOI: 10.1590/S1413-81232011000500031

[54] Alves YDD. O uso do crack como ele é: O cachimbo, o "bloco" e o usuário. Etnográfica. 2016;**20**:495-515. DOI: 10.4000/etnografica.4640

[55] Monteiro MG, Iniciardi JA, editors. Crack Cocaine in the Americas. São Paulo: Cebrid; 1993

[56] Bastos FI, Cotrim BC. O consumo de substâncias psicoativas entre os jovens brasileiros: Dados, danos e algumas propostas. In: JOVENS acontecendo na trilha das políticas públicas. Brasília: CNPD; 1998. pp. 645-670

[57] Zaluar A. Integração perversa: Pobreza e tráfico de drogas. Rio de Janeiro: Editora da Fundação Getúlio Vargas; 2004. 445 p. ISBN: 978-85-225-1986-6

[58] Sapori LF, Medeiros R, editors. Crack: Um desafio social. Belo Horizonte: Ed. PUC Minas; 2010. 220 p. ISBN: 978-85-60778-70-6

[59] Ribeiro LA, Sanchez ZM, Nappo SA. Strategies developed by crack users to deal with the risks resulting from the consumption. Jornal Brasileiro de Psiquiatria. 2010;**59**:210-218. DOI: 10.1590/S0047-20852010000300007

[60] Gonçalves JR, Nappo SA. Factors that lead to the use of crack cocaine in combination with marijuana in Brazil: A qualitative study. BMC Public Health. 2015;**15**:706. DOI: 10.1186/s12889-015-2063-0

[61] Almeida RBF. O caminho das pedras: Cultura de uso de crack em Pernambuco. Renata Barreto Fernandes de Almeida [thesis]. São Paulo: Federal University of São Paulo; 2017

[62] Santos NTV. Vulnerabilidade e prevalência de HIV e sífilis em usuários de drogas, Recife, 2009: Resultados de um estudo respondente-drivensampling [thesis]. Recife: Research Center Aggeu Magalhães—FIOCRUZ; 2013

[63] Santos NTV, Almeida RBF, Brito AM. Vulnerabilidade de usuários de crack a HIV e outras doenças transmissíveis: Estudo sóciocomportamental e de prevalência no estado de Pernambuco. Recife: Research Center Aggeu Magalhães—FIOCRUZ; 2016

[64] Diehl A, Cordeiro DC, Laranjeira R, editors. Dependência Química: Prevenção, Tratamento e Políticas Públicas. Porto Alegre: Artes Médicas; 2009. 528 p. ISBN: 978-85-363-2452-4

[65] Rodrigues VS, Horta RL, Szupszynski KPDR, Souza MC, Oliveira MS. Systematic review of psychological treatments for problems related to crack. Jornal Brasileiro de Psiquiatria. 2013;**62**:208-216. DOI: 10.1590/S0047-20852013000300005

[66] Petitjean SA, Dürsteler-MacFarland KM, Krokar MC, Strasser J, Mueller SE, Degen B, et al. A randomized, controlled trial of combined cognitive-behavioral therapy plus prize-based contingency management for cocaine dependence. Drug and Alcohol Dependence. 2014;**145**:94-100. DOI: 10.1016/j.drugalcdep.2014.09.785

[67] Araújo MR, Laranjeira R, editors. O Tratamento do usuário de crack. Porto Alegre: Artmed; 2012. 664 p. ISBN: 978-85-363-2631-3

[68] López-Torrecillas F, López-Quirantes EM, Maldonado A, Albein-Urios N, Rueda MDM, Verdejo-Garcia A. Decisional balance and processes of change in community-recruited with moderate-high versus mild severity of cannabis dependence. PLoS One. 2017;**12**:e0188476. DOI: 10.1371/journal.pone.0188476

[69] Romanini M, Dias ACG, Pereira AS. Grupo de prevenção de recaídas como dispositivo para o tratamento da dependência química. Disc Scientia. 2010;**11**:115-132. ISSN: 21773335

[70] Schneider JA, Limberger J, Andretta I. Habilidades sociais e drogas: Revisão sistemática da produção científica nacional e internacional. Avances en Psicología Latinoamericana. 2016;**34**:339-350. ISSNe: 2145-4515

[71] Oliveira GC, Nasi C, Lacchini AJB, Schneider JA, Pinho LB. Characteristics of work and strategies in mental health care with crack user. Enfermería Global. 2017;**47**:260-269. ISSN: 1695-6141

[72] Oliveira W. Psychiatric reform and psychosocial care in Brazil: Sociohistorical contextualization, challenges and perspectives. Brazilian Journal of Mental Health. 2012;**4**:52-71. ISSN: 2595-2420

[73] Guerra MRSR, Vandenberghe L. Abordagem do comportamento de uso abusivo de substâncias psicoativas no Brasil: O estado da arte. Pesquisas e Práticas Psicossociais. 2018;**13**:1-22. ISSN: 1809-8908

[74] Marchand WR. Mindfulness-based stress reduction, mindfulness-based cognitive therapy, and Zen meditation for depression, anxiety, pain, and psychological distress.

Journal of Psychiatric Practice. 2012;**18**:233-352. DOI: 10.1097/01.pra.0000416014.53215.86

[75] Marcus MT, Zgierska A. Mindfulness-based therapies for substance use disorders: Part 1 (editorial). Substance Abuse. 2009;**30**:263. DOI: 10.1080/08897070903250027

[76] Vásquez-Dextre ER. Mindfulness: Conceptos generales, psicoterapia y aplicaciones clínicas. Revista de Neuro-Psiquiatría. 2016;**79**:42-51. ISSN: 0034-8597

[77] Queiroz IS. Os programas de redução de danos como espaços de exercício da cidadania dos usuários de drogas. Psicologia: Ciência e Profissão. 2001;**21**:2-15. DOI: 10.1590/S1414-98932001000400002

[78] Araújo ACC, Pires RR. Harm reduction in psychosocial care: Conceptions and professional experiences in a CAPS ad. Tempus, Actas de Saúde Coletiva. 2017;**11**:9-21. DOI: 10.18569/tempus.v11i3.1982

[79] Morin E. O método 4, as idéias. Porto Alegre: Editora Sulina; 1991. 319 p. ISBN: 978-85-205-0597-7

[80] Morin E. Ciência com Consciência. Rio de Janeiro: Bertrand Brasil; 1999. 268 p. ISBN: 852-86-057-95

[81] Morin E. Da necessidade de um pensamento complexo. In: Martins FM, Silva JM, editors. Para navegar no século XXI: Tecnologias do Imaginário e Cibercultura. Porto Alegre: EdiPUCRS; 2000. pp. 19-42. ISBN: 852-05-021-99

[82] Maturana H, Paredes V, Magro C, editors. Cognição, ciência e vida cotidiana. Belo Horizonte: UFMG; 2001. 221 p. ISBN: 978-85-423-0027-7

[83] Maturana H, Magro C. Emoções e linguagem na educação e na política. Belo Horizonte: UFMG; 2005. 98 p. ISBN: 978-85-704-1152-5

[84] Maturana H. Self-consciousness: How? When? Where? Constructivist Foundations 1. 2006;**3**:91-102

[85] Rameh-de-Albuquerque RC. Da pessoa que recai à pessoa que se levanta: A recursividade dos que usam crack [thesis]. São Paulo: Federal University of São Paulo; 2017

[86] Cruz VD, Santos SSC, Gautério-Abreu DP, Silva BT, Ilha S. Drug consumption among elderly and harm reduction: A reflection from the complexity. Escola Anna Nery. 2016;**20**:e20160076. DOI: 10.5935/1414-8145.20160076

[87] Nichols MP, Schwartz RC. Terapia familiar: Conceitos e métodos. Porto Alegre: Artmed; 2007. 524 p. ISBN: 978-85-363-0910-1

[88] Prette ZD, Prette AD. Psicologia das habilidades sociais: Terapia, educação e trabalho. Petrópolis: Vozes; 2009. 206 p. ISBN: 853-26-2142-2

[89] Maturana H, Varela F. A árvore do conhecimento. São Paulo: Palas Athena; 2001. 288 p. ISBN: 857-24-2032-0

[90] Neil M, Silveira DX. Drogas e Redução de Danos: Uma cartilha para profissionais de saúde. UNIFESP, Ministério da Saúde: São Paulo; 2008. 96 p

Chapter 4

Neuroscience-Based Anthropological Psychiatry (NBAP): Ten Introductory Concepts

Martin L. Vargas

Abstract

Medicine can be done at very different levels. So, physical, biochemical, biological, and social medicine are disciplines that count with a large theoretical background. This multilevel approach is applicable to psychiatry too. The 1990s of the twentieth century was "The Decade of the Brain." It helped to conceive psychiatry as "biological psychiatry" in a mechanistic reductionist epistemology that has become the canonical paradigm for the speciality. But this perspective came across a problem. Psychiatric facts were defined in subjective terms, while the proposed models for this type of pathology were expressed attending to biological mechanisms without clear interlevel constructs for establishing associations between biology and subjective experiences or behavioral patterns. Although symptoms are subjective in a radical manner, associations do not appear in this way. Some kind of "incommensurability" appears between what we want to explain and the arguments we propose to. The price paid for the "hard objective" approximation of biological psychiatry is to replace subjective pathological experiences with mere objective indicators of them. In this chapter, we propose an alternative epistemological strategy by relying on "philosophically-oriented phenomenological psychopathology" (POPP) for the rigorous study of pathological subjectivity. A neuroscience-based anthropological psychiatry (NBAP) built on ten concepts is introduced.

Keywords: psychiatry, philosophical anthropology, phenomenology, philosophy of psychiatry, neurophenomenology, semantics

1. Introduction: the roots of the "philosophically-oriented phenomenological psychopathology"

In the last four decades, three paradigms deserve to be highlighted as models to be applied for the mental disorders.

The first one was diagnostic and statistical manual of mental disorders, third edition (DSM-III), emerging in the 1980s of the past century. It represented a nosological perspective which tried to be compatible with various other models (i.e. psychological, sociological) in addition to the medical one. Further actualizations of the DSM classification arrived at its last version, DSM-V, in 2013. The

International Classification of Diseases (ICD), at present in its 11th edition, corresponds, in essence, with DSM regarding to mental disorders.

The DSM was inspired in the Research Diagnostic Criteria of Robert Spitzer and other "neo-Kraepelinians," who tried to operationalize some subjective pathological experiences they obtained from the classical psychiatric nosology. DSM had a logical positivistic inspiration with the intention of being neutral about the postulated mechanisms for mental disorders. It is believed that the philosopher of science Carl Hempel influenced in the conception of DSM [1], but his true influence is now being discussed [2]. However, DSM supposed a determined attempt to operationalize the clinical work of the tradition that transits from Kraepelin to Jaspers and Schneider [3]. Kurt Schneider, as the main referent of the Heidelberg school, received the French and German tradition of the classical psychiatry and transferred this knowledge to the United Kingdom after World War II. The role played by Wilhelm Mayer-Gross in this tradition exportation to the Anglo-Saxon area was definitive [4].

Jaspers' General Psychopathology is undoubtedly the foundational text of theoretical psychiatry, namely psychopathology. But, although it is frequently argued that with this text phenomenology was introduced in psychopathology, the Husserlian method had less influence in Jaspers' thinking when compared with the impact that the differentiation between explaining and understanding of Dilthey had. Therefore, the Jasperian-Schneiderian psychopathology that inspired DSM should not be considered as radically phenomenological in Husserlian terms. Rather, the Jasperian theory proposes a methodological pluralism [5, 6] that bets for a psychopathological analysis that simultaneously explains and understands the complexity of any mental symptom. That complexity is mentioned by Mayer-Goss when writing on the diagnosis of schizophrenia in 1938 [7]:

"In psychological medicine we cannot proceed, as in general medicine, by collecting signs and symptoms and fitting them into a sort of jig-saw puzzle. All the symptoms have to be related to the psychological background against which they appear."

Neutrality was one of the main strengths of the DSM model. But it was turned into the focus of many critics in the last two decades, as DSM was vulnerable to manipulation by economic interests. Criticism against DSM has markedly increased over its successive editions [1]. The suspicion of fabricating spurious diseases which could be meaty objectives for the pharmaceutical market severely threatened the scientific value of DSM in the twenty-first century. Hence, nowadays, the idea that DSM is over has taken root.

As a response to the critics to DSM based on its epistemic vulnerabilities, a second paradigm has been trying to be implanted since 2008: The Research Domain Criteria project (RDoC). RDoC is an initiative of the National Institute of Mental Health (NIMH), first led by Thomas Insel, director of the NIMH. This initiative proposes to "develop, for research purposes, new ways of classifying mental disorders based on dimensions of observable behaviour and neurobiological measures" [8].

DSM classification is categorical and uses operationalization of subjective experiences. RDoC, on the other hand, differs from DSM in three main points: (1) RDoC proposes the use of dimensions instead of categories, (2) RDoC orients the core of the model toward domains or constructs with neurocognitive validity, abandoning the priority of interrater reliability that is a characteristic in DSM, and (3) RDoC intends to be a useful tool for research rather than a disease classificatory system. The change made from DSM-ICD model to the RDoC paradigm in the last decade has been characterized as an Aristotelian to Galilean turn. The DSM classification, which reifies mental disorders as natural categories of diseases (the Aristotelian perspective), has been substituted by the RDoC point of view, where biological and neurocognitive domains compound the matrix around which projecting new research programs (the Galilean perspective) [9].

Third, a phenomenological-based paradigm begins with the first years of the twenty-first century by the hand of Parnas and Zahavi [10] and other psychopathologists, which were hardly ascribed to the phenomenology of Edmund Husserl and who claim for an explicit philosophical foundation for psychopathology. They differentiate three uses of the term "phenomenology." The first one is that of the contemporary Anglo-Saxon psychiatric use, referring "phenomenology" to the mere "description of signs and symptoms of mental disorders." A second meaning would be the more restrictive use of the term in Jaspers, where phenomenology is "a study of inner experience." Finally, the third use of the term, the one Parnas and Zahavi defend, is the "endeavor inspired by phenomenological philosophy." Three are the most significant philosophers in this tradition, whose main texts were published over the middle years of the twentieth century: Edmund Husserl, Martin Heidegger, and Maurice Merleau-Ponty [11]. To disambiguate between the three uses of the term "phenomenology" in psychiatry, we will refer to this third meaning as "philosophically-oriented phenomenological psychopathology" (POPP), which constitutes, from our point view, the paradigm closer to an anthropological foundation of psychiatry.

Notice that POPP takes consciousness as the core function of the human brain functioning and that it is in consciousness where the psychopathological facts occur. POPP is, therefore, close to the "organo-dynamic theory" of mental illness of the French psychiatrist Henry Ey [12] as well as to Agustín Jimeno's "integral psychopathology," developed in Spain [13]. A kind of POPP has been extensively developed by Parnas et al. [11] around the psychopathology of schizophrenia, leading to the development of new instruments as EASE. Examination of anomalous self-experience (EASE) is a checklist for semi-structured, phenomenological exploration of subtle aspects of consciousness experience, described by Huber, Gross, Süllwold, Klosterkötter, and others [14] in the prodromal phase of schizophrenia. A second instrument, examination of anomalous world experience (EAWE) [15], has been recently developed by Sass and others with the same POPP orientation as EASE. In the case of EAWE, the exploration is not oriented to the inner space of the self, but to the outer world. Although EAWE was developed to be used in schizophrenic populations, it can be applied to other types of clinical groups too.

Organo-dynamic theory, integral psychopathology, EASE, and EAWE are four examples of the "Philosophically-Oriented Phenomenological Psychopathology" (POPP) we want to defend as a good model of psychopathology, which is coherent with anthropology. POPP will be the theoretical base of an anthropological psychiatry.

These are the four attributes that, in our perspective, characterize POPP: consciousness, phenomenology, semantics, and disintegration of semantics.

1. Consciousness: Consciousness is the dynamically structured global integrative function of the human being. Consciousness is the higher order homeostatic function of the human biology in an intersubjective social environment.

2. Phenomenology: The phenomenological method, first described by Husserl and later developed by Heidegger, Merleau-Ponty, and others, is a good philosophical method to the rigorous study of consciousness. The hermeneutical phenomenology of Heidegger [16] has interesting developments in psychotherapy [17]. Neurophenomenology, based in Merleau-Ponty's work, is applicable to neuroscience-oriented research of consciousness [18].

3. Semantics: Consciousness is a system composed of elements characterized to be meaning carrying entities. Following Fuster [19], we will name "cognit"

every element of the consciousness which is the minimal unit of semantics and that corresponds to a neural network. Cognits have mental properties in terms of the "psicons" as proposed by Bunge [20, 21]. Cognits are the element, both of conscious thinking and of language. Therefore, sharing equivalent cognits is the base for common sense or semantics in language and for intersubjectivity.

4. Disintegration of semantics: It is the key concept in psychopathology. Either in the personal attribution of relevance and significance to every cognit in the frame of a meaningful consciousness state, in an intersubjective dialog, or in a significant behavior, the elements of the consciousness must be capable of being integrated under a hermeneutically global sense. In the opposite case, the semantics of that conscious state can be denoted as psychopathological, lacking semantics, or senseless.

2. Neuroscience-based anthropological psychiatry

2.1 From POPP to NBAP

Once we have argued why to use a concrete psychopathological model, the POPP, and which are the four main attributes that characterizes it, two considerations must be explained: (1) its relationship whit the other mentioned psychopathological models and (2) its usefulness in anthropological psychiatry.

First, POPP is compatible with both DSM-ICD and RDoC models. POPP explores subtle aspects of consciousness experience, while DSM-ICD refers to unspecific verbal informs or to behavioral patterns. So POPP can be subsumed by DSM-ICD model, even though POPP aims to be a more exact and specific model while DSM-ICD sacrifices psychopathological fineness in favor of a massive epidemiological use. Although POPP and RDoC have different foundations (phenomenological the first and scientific positivist the second), its core constructs can be jointly studied under a correlational perspective. This is, precisely, the method that neurophenomenology proposes. The first-person perspective (or subjective phenomenological perspective) and the zero-person perspective (or objective scientific natural perspective) are both the dual approaching to any cognit. The neurophenomenological correlation makes the integration of both perspectives possible. This question will be further discussed at point 2.2.5. Note that in Anglo-Saxon literature, it is common to refer to the "zero-person perspective" as "third-person perspective." We prefer the term "zero-person" to denote that it is referred to an impersonal or objective (belonging to an object not a person) perspective. Phenomenological perspective in third person is not more than a first-person perspective after changing the ubication in the subjective space of the speaking subject to the subjective space of a third person. I thank the phenomenologist Javier San Martin for this observation on zero-person and third-person perspectives.

Second, we must aboard the question of why is POPP preferable for anthropological psychiatry or, in other words, why is anthropological psychiatry preferable for taking advantage of the phenomenological psychopathological tradition. The answer is that phenomenology is the philosophical foundation of both traditions: the psychopathological and the anthropological. Drawing from common sources will be the better guarantee for the consistence of the model.

The Spanish psychopathologist Demetrio Barcia defines anthropological psychiatry as the psychiatry which conceives that mental disease is an event that occurs in a human being ([22], p. 12). Following a perspective of philosophy of science, we have defined in a previous paper [13] anthropological psychiatry as the anthropological modeling of psychiatry. The first great incursion in this area was done by Ludwig Binswanger [23], and Otto Dörr has developed which is probably the most recent important systematic project of an explicit anthropological psychiatry [24]. Pelegrina [25, 26] makes a similar impressive recent work focusing not in psychiatry but in psychopathology. Once the former has been mentioned as paradigmatic examples, it is not our objective to systematically revise the many systems that can fall under the concept of anthropological psychiatry. We only want to point out that the majority, if not the totality of them, are before the conception of neurophenomenology as a bridge discipline between neuroscience and phenomenology. The model we propose, Neuroscience-Based Anthropological Psychiatry (NBAP), is an attempt to integrate recent neuroscience models in to the tradition of anthropological psychiatry.

The objective of this chapter, which will be developed in Section 2.2., is to present 10 concepts, introduced as 10 progressive steps, to characterize NBAP.

2.2 Ten introductory steps to NBAP

2.2.1 Phenomenology: the rigorous study of subjectivity

Modern science begins during the sixtieth and seventieth centuries by the leading hand of Galileo and Newton. The differentiation that Descartes did between res cogitans and res extensa facilitated the autonomy of empirical science from the philosophical speculation. The advance of the diverse scientific disciplines until the twentieth century gave rise to the idea that has been known as the spirit of Modernity. According to this, a unique objective reality exists. Its exact representation, preferably in mathematical terms, is the task of science. All the parcels of the unified science, from physics to psychology, must stick this presupposes if they want to be considered as scientific knowledge.

But, in the turn of nineteenth to twentieth centuries, a profound debate was sustained in the core of logic, psychology, and physics. The core of the problem was to delimitate what should be taken as the basic data of empiricism to construct any scientific argumentation. The discussion between Gottlob Frege and Edmund Husserl on the concept of number propitiated that the second began the way of phenomenology as the science of the essences. Phenomenology does not accept the idea that any mental concept is a representation of reality. Conversely, any mental content is the fact toward which the method of the phenomenological scientist must be oriented. "Back to the things themselves" was the slogan of Husserl and the phenomenological school in Germany in the first third of the twentieth century.

Phenomenology was the object of the critics of Rudolph Carnap and other philosophers of the science from the "Circle of Viena." Phenomenology was taken as an example of metaphysical nonsense, leading to a profound orientation in psychology toward facts nondependent on subjectivity, mainly the expressed behavior. The behavior observed in animals and humans under experimental conditions substitutes the mental experience as the focus of interest of most of the psychologists. In this context, which spread the central decades of the past century, the paradox occurred that scientific psychology took a rout while psychopathology remained inspired in the phenomenological origins of Jaspers and posteriorly the Heidelberg school. The picture complicates due to transactions between phenomenology and psychoanalysis that we cannot analyze here.

Phenomenological descriptions have been diverse in authors and perspectives over a great part of the past century. But this research was not placed at a central place in the academic psychiatry which, with the DSM-III era, evolved to a dominant biological mechanistic paradigm. It was during the turn to the present century when phenomenology was revisited and revaluated in the neuroscientific landscape [19] as well as in the psychopathological research [27]. Nowadays, a privileged circumstance allows us to reread the classical phenomenological descriptions. The umbrella of neuroscientist models allows us to subsume under them, at least in part, the classic phenomenology. The rigor of the descriptions of mental states in first person can be correlated with fine neurophysiological and neuroimage technics under common theoretical models. Moreover, the research program based on the topic of the mind as a black box has converged, via cognitive behaviors, to a renewed interest in mental events.

2.2.2 Phenomenological anthropology: the conditions of possibility of the human being

The question about the human being was one of the main challenges the modern thinking proposed. Kant was the enlightened thinker who, under the inspiration of Rousseau, initiated an explicit anthropological thinking. But the rational knowing on the human essence and its empirical characterization showed the difficulties and disadvantages consequent to applying the mechanistic models of the modern science to anthropological questions. Since the twentieth century, the anthropological inquires divide, between others, into three main streams: physical anthropology, cultural anthropology or ethnography, and philosophical anthropology.

Philosophical anthropology is the discipline we will focus on. Max Scheler, a philosopher who was initially ascribed to the Husserlian school, proposed for the first time the discipline in the 1920s of the twentieth century. After him, the discipline has become a philosophy of anthropology [28] in a similar way as a philosophy of psychology or a philosophy of medicine exists. But it is important to highlight a difference; while philosophy of medicine and philosophy of psychology mainly come from the analytical, positivistic, or Anglo-Saxon tradition in philosophy, philosophy of anthropology relates to the continental or phenomenology hermeneutical tradition. Nonetheless, currently both traditions are quickly mixing and enriching each other.

So, in the dotation of NBAP we have, now, phenomenology as a method for the rigorous study of subjectivity and philosophical anthropology as a framework in which to locate the empirical research regarding the human being. In this context, three specific questions can be done: (1) does the human condition change when sick? (2) which are the specific anthropological attributes of being a mentally ill person? and (3) how does the philosophy of the human being resolve the mind-brain and the identity-body problems? Further, these three questions will be addressed.

2.2.3 Anthropological medicine: a sick man and a doctor in a narrative circle

Medicine as we know it was born in essence with Hippocrates and his school on the fifth century BC. Before that time, medical practice touched the magical thinking and did not clearly differentiate from religion. But with Hippocratic medicine, disease, therapeutics, and the sick person-physician relationship changed to be inspired in the two complementary concepts of isonomy and philanthropy. The first of these concepts indicates that every citizen in Athens was equal under the law. The second principle, that specifically takes the form of medical philía [29], complements the former by virtue of helping others to achieve and to enjoy the condition of citizenship and, specifically, helping them to recover their health by means of medical science and art. Moreover, the ancient Greek cities stipulated the manutention of a physician in each one of them to protect the health of its inhabitants.

Although it seems obvious that modern medicine differs in many aspects from the ancient Greek medicine, mainly due to scientific and technological advances, we want to highlight that the core of it persists over the years since the times of Hippocrates. This core of the medical fact is no other than the patient-physician relationship.

After the scientific development of medicine that took place with the development of the clinic method in the university hospitals of the nineteenth century, medicine became a technical-scientific discipline even more, eclipsing its nuclear interpersonal essence. But the work of Freud and its followers was a revulsive to the very modern perspective of the medicine that predominated during the positivist attitude of the second half of the nineteenth century. With Freud, the patient-physician relationship turns to the focus of medicine, now under the name of "transference."

It is around this rescued reality of intersubjectivity in medicine where the anthropological medicine of Viktor von Weizsäcker should be considered [30, 31]. The work of Viktor von Weizsäcker is mainly located at Heidelberg in the 1930s–1950s of the past century. He was a doctor, specialist in internal medicine and in neurology as well as a philosopher whose original thinking was inspired by psychoanalyzes, phenomenology, and philosophical anthropology. von Weizsäcker stressed that the sick person has a biography the doctor must take in account to the rigorous understanding of the where, when, what, and why of any disease. This anthropological perspective is not opposite, but complementary, with the technical-scientific one. The integration of both perspectives led to a global comprehension of the sickness condition. The "pathic" dimension of the human being (the emotional nonconscious coming from the body) integrates with the "ontic" one (the rational conscious coming from the rational mind) in a circle of Gestalt or configuration (Gestaltkreis). This configurative circle unifies both the "solidarity of death" and the "reciprocity of life" in a way that radically includes disease and death with health and life, remarking the idea that sickness is consubstantial to the human being. In this scene, the role of the physician far to "fight against the death" is "pact with the death." After von Weizsäcker, the patient-physician relationship has been profoundly theorized by Laín Entralgo [29].

The patient-physician relationship has become the axis or nuclear construct around which present medical theory is constructed. From a reification of diseases as mere natural regularities remaining at the center of a play where the doctor is the active agent while the patient passively remains as "the land where the battle takes place," contemporary medicine has evolved to a "narrative dialog" [32]. Patient and physician now dialog and jointly assume risks and take decisions considering the data provided by evidence-based knowledge. We are in an ethical context of autonomy and responsibility [33], not yet in the paternalism that accompanied the mechanistic medicine of the "diseases as natural species." Anthropological medicine will undoubtedly help in the construction of the dialogic intersubjective patient-physician relationship which present medicine claims for.

2.2.4 Anthropological psychiatry: medicine of the subjectivity

The phenomenological anthropological perspective in medicine has been intensively applied in psychiatry [34]. Ludwig Binswanger, a Swedish psychiatrist contemporary of von Weizsäcker, integrates in his "existential analysis" [23] some aspects of the psychoanalytical tradition for the analysis of the Dasein, the construct that subsumes the human being under the point of view of the Heideggerian hermeneutical phenomenology. Many psychiatrists followed the trail that Binswanger initiated in his application of philosophical anthropology to psychiatry.

Wolfgang Blankenburg applied the phenomenological analysis under a Husserlian perspective to the self-experience of schizophrenia. He proposed that the phenomenological key of this condition is the "loss of the natural evidence" in relation with the world [35]. Hubertus Tellenbach, applying the phenomenological method, described the "Typus melancholicus" that he characterizes by order attachment, strong moral conscience, intolerance to the ambiguity, and hypernomy-heteronomy. These phenotypical traits would predispose to endogenous depression.

Many other original proposes were done mainly in the German area, which located the very different ways the Heideggerian Dasein has to be in the world. These fine observations of the very different modes that the human existence has for expressing himself progressively erased the frontier between "normality" and mental illness. Outside the German area, in his classical book "The divided self" [36], the Scottish psychiatrist Ronald Laing finally proposed to solve that frontier doing comprehensible the madness using the method of the existential analysis. The barriers had been demolished, and the antipsychiatry arguments were knocking on the door whipped by Foucault.

From Binswanger to Foucault, medical anthropology embarked on a trip after which the classical image of the human being, and, also, his existential reformulation, arrived at a postmodern subject who will be progressively diluted in language and the social structure to definitively arrive to Lacan. This transgression is enough to illustrate the very diverse ways that the anthropological map can conduct the contemporary conception of the human being as a subject.

2.2.5 Neurophenomenology: the world-brain-mind system

The "naturalization of phenomenology" [37] became a new topic with the diffusion of the French philosopher Maurice Merleau-Ponty's works in the second half of the twentieth century. His theory propitiated "the body turn" of phenomenology, placing the human body at the center of the perception of the world. But not only the body as the lived axis of the world but the body, and more exactly the brain in its relationship with consciousness and subjectivity, has been taking center stage in the philosophical anthropology of the new millennium.

This naturalization and turn to the brain have implicated the broad territory of philosophy of the mind. In the analytical tradition, this reorientation has resulted in the concept of "neurophilosophy," led by the philosophers Patricia and Paul Churchland [38]. As a response, or a complement, the neuroscientist and phenomenologist Francisco Varela proposed in 1996 the concept of "neurophenomenology" [18, 39], by which he wanted to tackle the "hard problem" of consciousness. In his seminal work [18], Varela clarifies:

"the Working Hypothesis of Neurophenomenology: Phenomenological accounts of the structure of experience and their counterparts in cognitive science relate to each other through reciprocal constraints."

Complementary to the construct of neurophenomenology, Varela proposed a second fundamental concept: "enaction." It implies a deep reconceptualization of problems being classically addressed by the cognitive sciences, so that enaction can be taken as a serious alternative to the concept of representative cognition. Writes Varela [37], p. 272:

"My overall approach to cognition is based on situated, embodied agents. I have introduced the name enactive to designate this approach more precisely. It comprises two complementary aspects: (1) the ongoing coupling of the cognitive agent, a permanent coping that is fundamentally mediated by sensorimotor activities; and (2) the autonomous activities of the agent whose identity is based on emerging, endogenous configurations (or self-organizing patterns) of neuronal activity.

Enaction implies that sensorimotor coupling modulates, but does not determine, an ongoing endogenous activity that it configures into meaningful world items in an unceasing flow."

As we can see, the idea of self-organization of the mind processes reappears in Varela in a similar way we saw when mentioning the Gestaltkreis in von Weizsäcker. Self-organization of mind processes appear as a key concept too in the model proposed by another seminal author we want to mention: Joaquín M. Fuster. In his book of 2003, Cortex and Mind [19], Fuster introduces two concepts which can be very helpful to a neuroscience-based anthropological psychiatry: the cognit and the perception-action cycle. This is how Fuster defines both ideas:

"To characterize the cognitive structure of a cortical network, I use the term cognit, a generic term for any representation of knowledge in the cerebral cortex. A cognit is an item of knowledge about the world, the self, or relations between them." (p. 14).

"Earlier I alluded to long connections from posterior cortical areas to areas of the frontal lobe. These connections constitute the functional linkage between the two cortical hierarchies, one for perception in posterior cortex and the other for action in frontal cortex. The lowest stages of both hierarchies are the cortical processing areas at the interface between the cortex and the environment: sensory cortex at the input interface and motor cortex at the output interface. In the course of behaviour, the two hierarchies are engaged in a cybernetic cycle of dynamic interactions with the environment that I have termed the perception-action cycle". (p. 74).

"The cognitive interactions of a primate with the surrounding world are governed by what I have named the perception-action cycle [40]. This interactive cycle is the extension to cortical processes of a basic principle of biology that characterizes the dynamic adaptation of an organism to its environment. It was first proposed by the biologist Uexküll [41], who deduced it from behavioral observations in a large number of animal species. Essentially, it can be stated as follows. An animal's behavior consists of a succession of adaptative motor reactions to changes in its external and internal environments." (pp. 107–108).

To summarize the approximation to NBAP we are doing from Sections 2.2.1 to 2.2.5, anthropology is the discipline that specifically studies the human being. It needs to achieve symbolic facts, which are presented as subjective mental states. The rigorous study of the mental states implies accounting for the system composited by the human animal, its historical and cultural narrative, and the intersubjective and physical medium where he or she lives. By "rigorous study," we mean both the explication and the comprehension. "Elucidating" could be a term that includes both significances. Different traditions termed diversely this system: Gestalkrise, perception-action system, hermeneutics. They are not synonymous terms, but they share an attribute definitory of the living things: self-organization or in the Maturana's classical term "autopoiesis." So the human being is an autopoietic system composited by symbolic elements (namely, semantic elements or cognits). This fragile system emerges in a concrete cultural and physical environment with which the person makes semantic and physical transactions to the moment of its disintegration due to death. Medical processes are those where a high risk of disintegration exists. Psychiatric processes, for its part, are those where the risk of disintegration mainly appears in the semantic aspects of the system.

The philosopher of science Mario Bunge proposes a scientific metaphysical [42] system based, among others, on the concept of "system." Following the ontology of Bungean's scientific metaphysics, we propose that a human being is the system characterized by the following: (1) Its "components" are cognits, which we define as neural networks self-poetically emerging; (2) the "environment" of any human system is the semiotic context where it develops; (3) cognits dynamically stabilize by virtue of biological "mechanisms" needed by the whole integrity of the body to maintain its fragile integrity; and (4) the "structure" of a human system is in part common to all the human beings (see below "the personal matrix") while it is in part idiosyncratic as well (personal character or self-identity). Note that (3) refers to neurobiology, (1) to semantics, (2) is related with linguistics, and (4) corresponds to philosophical anthropology. This ontology satisfies what García [43] proposes for any theoretical model designed to be applicable to complex systems, which must be compatible with different scientific disciplines. So defining a human being as a kind of system facilitates our objective with respect to NBAP, as the model is applicable to the anthropological processes targeted as "normal," "physiological," or "ethnographic" as well as to the other that tradition qualifies as "pathological." In other work, we propose a similar systemic approach to the problem of putatively defining humanity in artificial systems [44]. In our view, basing neurophenomenology in Bunge's scientific ontology implies a significant advantage over which modeling NBPA.

2.2.6 *The personal matrix: mapping subjectivity*

The great majority of people share a conjunct of attributes or dimensions that can be accepted as "universals" in the human being. Every person can be ascribed to a numeric or categorical value in the attributes of age, gender, language, or ethnic group. These four attributes would be ethnographic axes as a part of a personal matrix that could count with multiple other dimensions.

The ethnographic or "cultural universals" just mentioned are easy to apprehend in a first approximation to the problem. But the phenomenological work really begins when we try to extract the common subjective dimensions that "transcendentally" structures human systems in people from different cultures and epochs. This is what might be called "positive or empirical phenomenological research." To illustrate this idea, following a canonical text [45], we can mention some classical dimensions, axes, or topics in phenomenology each one of those could be a dimension of the personal matrix: that is, bodily intentionality, self-consciousness and world-consciousness, epistemic commonality and truth, or time experience.

In other work [46], we defined a matrix composed by eight phenomenological dimensions (four related with time and four related with space) and four limits to the phenomenological experience. The time dimensions are as follows: morality, the ongoing task, desire, and hope. Every one of these dimensions can be explored when we try to "anthropologically elucidate" a person. Morality is the system of behavioral patterns that constitute us before any intentional act. The task ongoing is the one that makes me feel an intentional subject. Desire is a behavioral pattern at present activated but still not closed in a perception-action cycle. Hope is a behavioral pattern I recognize as desirable but presently inactive. The space dimensions are the body as entrails, the body as flesh, circumstance, and landscape. Body as entrails is the experience of the emotional response of the body (anger, joyfulness, and so on). Body as flesh refers to the experience of the body as the organism that accompanies my biographical live and where my subjectivity is embodied. Circumstance is the environment composed by the other people and by the artificial objects I interact with in my present intentional acts. The landscape is composed by the living beings and inorganic materials I can see or imagine but with which I am not at present interacting and which stay as a mere environment of my lived experience. The four limits of the phenomenological experience are death, absence, self, and mind.

A rich phenomenological elucidation is documented of any of these and much other similar phenomenological concepts. The positive work of the phenomenologist community from Husserl to date is the rigorous description of the fabric over which the structure of the human being emerges, as well as the very different characteristic variants that it takes in every individual person. Additionally, a priority for the near future would be to establish correlations between the main phenomenological concepts and the intrinsic connectivity brain networks [47]. Attending to a neurophenomenological framework, a desirable research agenda in neurophenomenology would be to describe the personal phenomenological matrix in terms of visual (landscape), somatomotor (ongoing task), dorsal attention (circumstance), ventral attention (morality, desire, and hope), limbic (body as entrails), frontoparietal (body as flesh), default (self and mind).

2.2.7 Semantics: sharing personal fields

"The mind is intentional," affirms a topic of the phenomenology coming from the pre-Husserlian days of Brentano. Every subjective experience has an object toward which the mind is projected. In a perception-action cycle, the motor system is projected to the world, executing an intentional plan. When two or more people share an objective, they form a system and share a global intentional motor plan. So, the association of this intentional motor plan to a motor verbal behavior is facilitated while a verbal sound appears in the common circumstance of the group.

The verbal sound becomes a new component of that shared circumstance, with a relevant characteristic: as well as the visual perspective changes profoundly from each of the persons implicated in the common task, the sound involves the perceptual field of every component of the group equally. So, this sound, that is closely associated to the vital fact in course, becomes commonly significant. The sound acquires meaning with the result that a verbal sign emerges.

The shared pragmatic field derives in a shared sign that, finally, constitutes a shared ontology by the linguistic nature of the human mind. Precisely, it is due to the common transcendental structure that we humans share that the shared pragmatic and semantic fields can become a common ontology. This common ontology is no other than the "common sense."

Every culture and epoch has a common sense, whose components are group's shared pragmatic fields. They constitute the ontology, the semantic base of their language, in other words: the reality for that human group.

2.2.8 Mental signs: aliens in the common sense

The medical rationality has constructed the conceptual object of "disease." A disease is a component of the pragmatic field, at list in contemporary occidental human groups. The infective diseases conformed the classical paradigm of diseases, which Thomas Sydenham in seventieth century contributes to fix as "natural species." So, disease is a reified conceptual object that the physician tries to perceive and recognize looking for several physical, laboratory, radiological, or biological indices. In the classical clinical theory, a sign is a data obtained in the clinical exploration that means that a disease can be present.

Since psychiatry is a medical speciality, it shares the method that looks for signs of diseases. But, in this case, the signs come not from the visual, tactile, or sound perception. The psychiatrist detects signs by a method that, somehow, "perceives" the mental subjectivity of the patient through the enquiry for a sense in the motor and verbal behavior of the patient in a concrete context. The sharing of a common sense between a psychiatrist and a patient coming from the same language community, culture, and epoch, makes it possible to detect mental states which are "out from the shared field of the common sense." When it is supposed that it is because a body disease exists, affecting the mechanism of the mind, the psychiatrist judges that a psychiatric disease is present. When the psychiatrist, or the clinical psychologist, judges that the biological mechanism of the brain is normally functioning, even though the patient is out of the common sense, a psychiatric disorder without disease is present.

The concept of mental sign is necessary if we accept that psychiatry is medicine. Clerambault's mental automatism is a classic example of that perspective. So, the main diagnostic task of the clinical psychiatrist is to detect the presence, or not, of several mental signs that lead to a diagnosis. In terms of Jaspers, the mental signs can be explained but cannot be understood. Therefore, we can characterize any mental sign as "xenopatic," namely "an alien" in the common sense.

2.2.9 The clinical neurophenomenological method: revisiting psychiatry

Taking in account Sections 2.2.1 to 2.2.8, in other work [46], we have proposed the technical steps to follow in the applying of the termed "clinical neurophenomenological method". It consists in:

1. To adopt a phenomenological matrix model:
    a. to adopt a system of temporal and space anthropological attributes;
    b. to adopt a system of brain's associative neural networks;
    c. to adopt a correlation's matrix between anthropological attributes and neural networks.
2. To define the personal field's matrix:
    a. to determine the concrete temporal attributes of the matrix in that patient;
    b. to determine the concrete special attributes of the matrix in that patient.
3. To reduce the symptom to a lived experience:
    a. focalizing the symptom in zero-person;
    b. reducing the symptom to lived experience by adopting in second-person perspective of the patient;
    c. placing the lived experience in the correspondent cell at the personal matrix.
4. Understanding analyses of the lived experience:
    a. to active, by means of introspection, the correspondent cell in the phenomenologist's personal field;
    b. to empathically understand the lived experience in first-person;
    c. contrasting with the patient the sense of the lived experience;
    d. replacing in the matrix the lived experience, if necessary, attending to the new information after contrasting the information with the patient.

5. Psychopathological analyses:

   a. detecting positive mental signs;

   b. detecting negative mental signs;

   c. detecting secondary psychopathological organizers, which patients construct to stabilize his or her psychopathological system;

   d. to postulate the neural network which is implied in the positive and negative signs and, if the case, the subjacent brain connectivity pathology.

6. Therapeutic dialog:

   a. facilitating the mental sign's symbolization by means of a psychotherapeutic dialog;

   b. supporting the patient in the adaptative modulation of his or her psychopathological organizers;

   c. to propose new organizers in the personal field, which were based in the common sense.

2.2.10 Therapeutic dialog: back to the common sense

If mental signs are understandable, the task of psychotherapy is to cover these "alien to the self" experiences by a narrative which could be shared, at least, by two people: the patient and the psychotherapist. By the fact of being shared, the pathological experience begins to be covered by a "semantic covering."

Note that, then, the psychiatrist's task is double and bidirectional, as already pointed Jaspers with his methodological pluralism [5]. He or she must, as a physician, attend to the biologically explainable, but do not understandable, of the mental experience. Also, they, as a psychotherapist, must help in covering the experience of the patient with a unitary and shared sense. With this anthropological perspective, Giovanni Stanghellini [17] has developed a rigorous psychotherapeutic method we based in: the phenomenological hermeneutic dialectic (PHD) method, to which the reader is referred.

In view of the above, we can define in easy terms neuroscience-based anthropological psychiatry (NBAP) as a medical-psychotherapeutic specialty.

3. Conclusions

Psychiatry is a medical-psychotherapeutic speciality. In this chapter, it has been proposed that the psychotherapeutic dialog is the technique we can use to progressively cover with successive layers of common sense the alien mental signs that presents in the lived experience of the patient. This technique is complementary to the medical intervention of diagnose and pharmacological and physical treatment of the body diseases which affects the normal brain functioning. To the study of brain functioning, in addition to laboratory, neuroimage, and neurophysiological technics, the clinical neurophenomenologist uses the specific method of exploring the enactive functioning of the patient's brain. In this task, to achieve a shared semantics in the patient-physician anthropological encounter is necessary.

Medicine is a complex art. It needs the collaboration of the biological and social sciences. But a rigorous philosophical foundation is also necessary for psychiatry.

Conflict of interest

The author declares no conflict of interest.

Notes/thanks/other declarations

This chapter is part of the research program "Neurophenomenology: theory and critic for an anthropological foundation of psychiatry" included in the research line "Phenomenology, philosophical anthropology and philosophy of religion" of the Faculty of Philosophy, Universidad Nacional de Educación a Distancia (UNED), Spain.

Author details

Martin L. Vargas
University Hospital Rio Hortega, Valladolid University, Valladolid, Spain

*Address all correspondence to: mvargas@saludcastillayleon.es

References

[1] Decker HS. The Making of DSM-III: A Diagnostic manual's Conquest of American Psychiatry. Oxford: Oxford University Press; 2013

[2] Cooper R, Blashfield R. The myth of Hempel and the DSM-III. Studies in History and Philosophy of Biological and Biomedical Sciences. 2018;**70**:10-19

[3] Janzarik W. Jaspers, Kurt Schneider and the Heidelberg school of psychiatry. History of Psychiatry. 1998;**ix**:241-252

[4] De Leon J. "Es hora de despertar a la Bella Durmiente" En 1980, la psiquiatría europea cayó en un profundo sueño. Revista de Psiquiatría y Salud Mental. 2014;**7**:186-194

[5] Stanghellini G, Fuchs T, editors. One Century of Karl Jaspers' General Psychopathology. Oxford: Oxford University Press; 2013

[6] Huber G. The psychopathology of K. Jaspers and and K. Schneider as a fundamental method for psychiatry. The World Journal of Biological Psychiatry. 2002;**3**:50-57

[7] Mayer-Gross W. The early diagnosis of schizophrenia. British Medical Journal. 1938;**2**:936-939

[8] Cuthbert BN. The RDoC framework: Facilitating transition from ICD/DSM to dimensional approaches that integrate neuroscience and psychopathology. World Psychiatry. 2014;**13**:28-35

[9] Lilienfeld SO, Treadway MT. Clashing diagnostic approaches: DSM-ICD versus RDoC. Annual Review of Clinical Psychology. 2016;**12**:435-463

[10] Parnas J, Zahavi D. The role of phenomenology in psychiatric dignosis and classification. In: Maj M, Gaebel W, López-Ibor JJ, et al., editors. Psychiatric Diagnosis and Classification. West Sussex, UK: John Wiley & Sons, Ltd; 2002 [Epub ahead of print 2002]. DOI: 10.1192/bjp.113.500.765

[11] Parnas J, Møller P, Kircher T, et al. EASE: Examination of anomalous self-experience. Psychopathology. 2005;**38**:236-258

[12] Farina B, Ceccarelli M, Di Giannantonio M. Henri Ey's neojacksonism and the psychopathology of disintegrated mind. Psychopathology. 2005;**38**:285-290

[13] Vargas ML. Agustín Jimeno Valdés's integral psychopathology: Context and concepts. Neuroscience and History. 2018;**6**(3):74-84

[14] Schultze-Lutter F, Debbané M, Theodoridou A, et al. Revisiting the basic symptom concept: Toward translating risk symptoms for psychosis into neurobiological targets. Front Psychiatry. 2016;7 [Epub ahead of print 2016]. DOI: 10.3389/fpsyt.2016.00009

[15] Sass L, Pienkos E, Skodlar B, et al. EAWE: Examination of anomalous world experience. Psychopathology. 2017;**50**:10-54

[16] León EA. El giro hermenéutico de la fenomenológica en Martín Heidegger 2019. Available from: Polisjournals.openedition.org/polis/2690

[17] Stanghellini G. Lost in Dialogue. Anthropology, Psychopathology, and Care. Oxford: Oxford University Press; 2017

[18] Varela FJ. Neurophenomenology. A methodological remedy for the hard problem. Journal of Consciousness Studies. 1996;**3**:330-349

[19] Fuster JM. Cortex and Mind. Unifying Cognition. Oxford: Oxford University Press; 2003

[20] Bunge M. Materia y mente. Una investigación filosófica. Barcelona: Laetoli; 2015

[21] Vargas ML. Neurosciences and philosophy: What is new in the 21st century? Neuroscience and History. 2017;**5**:38-46

[22] Barcia D, editor. Psiquiatría antropológica. Homenaje al Profesor H. Tellenbach. Murcia: Universidad de Murcia; 1987

[23] Ghaemi SN. Rediscovering existential psychotherapy: The contribution of Ludwig Binswanger. American Journal of Psychotherapy. 2001;**55**:51-64

[24] Dörr O. Psiquiatría Antropológica. Contribuciones a una psiquiatría de orientación fenomenológico-antropológica. 3rd ed. Santiago de Chile: Editorial Universitaria; 2017

[25] Pelegrina Cetran H. Fundamentos Antropológicos de la Psicopatología. Madrid: Polifemo; 2006

[26] Pelegrina CH. Psicopatología regional. Estructuras dimensionales de la psicopatología. Logopatías y timopatías. Madrid: Polemos; 2017

[27] Gallagher S, Zahavi D. The Phenomenological Mind. London: Routledge; 2013

[28] Zirión QA. Prólogo para el libro 'Antropología y fenomenología (Tomo I)'. Investigaciones Fenomenológicas. 2015;**12**:209-220

[29] Laín EP. La relación médico-emfermo. Historia y teoría. Madrid: Revista de Occidente; 1964

[30] Weizsäcker V von. Der kranke Mensch. Eine Einführung in die medizinische Anthropologie. Stuttgart: Koheler; 1951

[31] Wiedebach H. Some aspects of a medical anthropology: Pathic existence and causality in Viktor von Weizsäcker. History of Psychiatry. 2009;**20**:360-376

[32] Charon R. Narrative medicine. A model for empathy, reflection, profession, and trust. JAMA. 2001;**286**:1897-1902

[33] Kilbride MK, Joffe S. The new age of patient autonomy implications for the patient-physician relationship. JAMA. [Epub ahead of print 2018]. DOI: 10.1001/jama

[34] Dörr Zegers O. La fenomenología psiquiátrica como epistemología y sus consecuencias terapéuticas. Revista de Neuro-Psiquiatría. 2005;**68**:3-15

[35] Der Blanckenburg W. Verlust der natürlichen Selbstverständlichkeit: Ein Beitrag zur Psychopathologie symptomarmer Schizophrenien. Parodos Verlag; 2012

[36] Laing R. The Divided Self: An Existential Study in Sanity and Madness. London: Penguin; 1990

[37] Petitot J, Varela FJ, Pachoud B, et al. Naturalizing Phenomenology. Stanford: Stanford University Press; 1999

[38] Churchland PS. Neurophilosophy. Toward a Unified Science of the Mind/Brain. Cambridge, Massachusetts: The MIT Press; 1986

[39] Varela FJ, Thompson E, Rosch E. The Embodied Mind. Cognitive Science and Human Experience. Cambridge, Massachusetts: The MIT Press; 1993

[40] Fuster JM. Memory in the Cerebral Cortex: An Empirical Approach to Neural Networks in the Human and Nonhuman Primate. Cambridge, MA: MIT Press; 1995

[41] Uexküll JV. Theoretical Biology. New York: Harcourt, Brace; 1926

[42] Bunge M. Is scientific metaphysics possible? Journal of Philosophy. 1971;**68**:507-520

[43] García R. Interdisciplinariedad y sistemas complejos. Rev Latinoam Metodol las Ciencias Soc. 2011;**1**:66-101

[44] Vargas AM. Inteligencia artificial versus inteligencia natural: Apuntes para una gnoseología de fundamentación antropológica. Kranion. 2019;**14**:24-30

[45] Zahavi D. The Oxford Handbook of Contemporary Phenomenology. Oxford: Oxford University Press; 2012

[46] Vargas AM. Neurofenomenología, enacción y cerebro: hacia una neurofenomenología clínica. Kranion. 2018;**13**:41-47

[47] Sporns O. Cerebral cartography and connectomics. Philosophical Transactions of the Royal Society B: Biological Sciences. 2015;**370**:1-12

Chapter 5

The Mental Health of Combatants

Andrey Soloviev, Elena Ichitovkina and Marina Zlokazova

Abstract

The chapter deals with the theoretical, methodological, and practical aspects of combatants' mental health as participants in hostilities, in the context of psychosocial environment characteristics and the transformation of personal characteristics in the process of stress service. The emerging situational and dynamic nosological and subclinical changes are described, which do not lead to social disintegration during the service. The study of the power structure of employees' catamnesis for 10 years of service was conducted with an assessment of social adaptation to peaceful life from clinical and psychological positions. The efficiency of complex therapy for persons with post-traumatic stress disorder and adaptation disorders is estimated, and the features of the organization of stage-by-stage rehabilitation with a team poly-professional approach are described. The methods allowing to predict the formation of borderline mental disorders (BMD) in this contingent are offered. The directions of medical and psychological support of combatants with the creation of a fundamentally new diagnostic, psychoprophylactic structure—the Center of Mental Health—to improve the quality of psychological and psychiatric care and monitoring of participants of the fighting mental state are systematized.

Keywords: combatants, borderline mental disorders, prevention, therapy, rehabilitation

1. Introduction

Preservation of mental health and extension of professional longevity of combatants are the most urgent task of departmental psychiatry, as they are the most important element of public health, largely determining the economic and social well-being of the nation.

When considering the mental health of combatants in the context of the characteristics of the psychosocial environment and the dynamics of personal characteristics in the process of stress service, many authors note the presence of situational and dynamic subclinical changes that do not lead to social maladaptation in the usual conditions (in the circle of colleagues) [16], but significantly worsen the family sphere of functioning and contribute to a decrease in the quality of life.

Issues of psychological prevention of the formation of borderline mental disorders (BMD) and destructive and addictive behavior of combatants come to the fore in their social and psychological significance: suicidal and antisocial actions, use of drugs, and alcohol abuse [5].

The structure of mental disorders in combatants in recent decades is characterized by a predominance of acute psychogenic pathological disorders with a significant reduction in the number of reactive psychosis. Over time, the structure of the social and medical consequences of wars for persons involved in extreme situation

(ES) begins to prevail in the BMD, which lead not only to a decrease in the quality of life but also premature disability [6].

Combatants' BMD are characterized by a wide range of mental illnesses from mild affective disorders and post-traumatic stress disorder (PTSD) to severe personality disorders.

The Russian army began fighting in the North Caucasus region (NCR) against the separatists on December 11, 1994—it was the most massive and brutal war in the history of modern Russia. On August 31, 1996, the fight ended with the signing of the Khasavyurt agreement. However, the end of the conflict did not bring peace and tranquility. Kidnappings and murders of people, terrorist attacks on the territory of Russia led to the second stage of the military confrontation with the need to involve professional employees—members of law enforcement agencies. Fighting clashes took place in the territory of some republics—Chechnya, Ingushetia, Dagestan, and Kabardino-Balkaria. According to the general staff of the armed forces of the Russian Federation, during the period of hostilities in 1994–2009, the irretrievable losses of the Russian security agencies in the North Caucasus amounted to killed and dead of more than 8500, prisoners and missing of 510, and wounded of more than 70,000 people.

The dynamics of personal changes in combatants indicates the deterioration of their mental health; there are emotional and behavioral stress, hyperactivity, a tendency to aggressive reactions, signs of social maladaptation, psychasthenic features, introversion, and emotional coldness, which contribute to the change of social functioning and social disintegration in the absence of clinically expressed psychopathology [14]. Therefore, it is necessary to detect these violations early and carry out medical and rehabilitation measures with subsequent monitoring of mental health of the participants of the fight.

2. Borderline mental disorders in combatants

Among the clinical forms of BMD, to identify the combatants, the most common are an organic disorder with personality disorders, affective disorders and organic mental syndrome (F06, F07 according to *ICD-10*), somatoform disorders (F45), PTSD (F43.1), adjustment disorders (F43.2), and chronic changes of personality after the experience of catastrophe (F62.0).

Combatants' BMD are significantly different from civilian neuroses on the specifics of the formation of the clinical symptoms and clinical manifestations; it is consistent with the formation of neurosis on the background of acquired and eventually increasing "accentuation of combatant" [17]. Earlier, the sudden onset of psychopathological symptoms was described against the background of external well-being, in acute conflict situations, often reflecting the internal feelings of a combatant [6].

From the point of view of S. Sukiasyan [14], BMD formed under the influence of combat mental trauma have similarities with neuroses in civilians. He distinguishes the following differences due to the etiopathogenesis of the disease and its dynamics: (a) the cause of the disease is characterized by an extreme occurrence, (b) the disorder occurs simultaneously from a large number of people, and (c) stress experienced by a person that is considered senseless leads to feelings of guilt for what happened with another person (death, injury, etc.).

According to M. Aksenov et al. [2], psychogenic neurotic states in persons of dangerous professions are presented by structured and relatively stable borderline disorders in their "classical" forms of manifestation (hysterical, dissociative, depressive, obsessive, anxiety-phobic, asthenic patterns, "neurosis of exhaustion").

A distinctive feature of combatants' BMD is the presence of an alcohol component, which is an integral part of the structure of mental disorders and before the formation of symptoms of dependence. In comorbid alcohol and drug disorders, there is no stage of formation of dependencies, in the structure of violations prevailing mainly psychopathic component. Drug dependence is more common among combatants who have had occasional drug use during fighting, who have not had sufficient socialization in peaceful life, and who had clinical signs of PTSD with a lack of timely treatment.

A special role among all combatants' BMD is given to PTSD. Psychotraumatic events of combat nature can lead to the formation of chronic forms of PTSD, often occurring exclusively at the subclinical level, while disrupting the social functioning and quality of life in the participants of the fight. The following clinical variants of anxiety, explosive, dysphoric, depressive, somatoform, and conversion are described [4].

Descriptions of the clinical picture of PTSD include polymorphic asthenic, obsessive-phobic, and anxiety-depressive symptoms. According to J.Alexander [1], rare fully phenomenologically defined clinical variants of PTSD, there is a tendency to combination with the socio-stress disorders.

Manifestations of post-traumatic stress disorder are often protracted, forming an average of 2–6 months after exposure to a traumatic situation. Personality disorders caused by battle mental trauma continue to be one of the most difficult areas of military psychiatry, both in clinical and diagnostic and in medical and expert aspects. Shortcomings in diagnostic approaches in the early stages lead to the identification of diseases at the stage of "deep implantation" of psychopathological symptoms in the personality, which later becomes the cause of the formation of pronounced personality disorders with subsequent disability of combatants.

Ignoring the symptoms of borderline mental disorders or their late detection, a formal approach by specialists in their diagnosis leads to the formation of chronic neurotic disorders, which significantly reduces the quality of life of combatants, increases the risk of manifestations of various forms of deviant behavior (antisocial, suicidal, addictive) [10].

To explore the mental health of combatants involved in fighting in the North Caucasus, a continuous survey of 1537 men—employees of power structures of Russia returned from the trip after the execution of service and combat tasks in the special conditions as a member of integrated fighting units in the period 2006–2009—was carried out. Among all surveyed on the level of mental health identified after participating in the hostilities, believable: (a) Seven hundred twenty-five persons (45.7%)—healthy combatants, whom the therapy was not required, and rehabilitation assistance was not provided. (b) Four hundred ninety-seven people (31.3%)—persons who for 6 years prior to the survey according to the data of the outpatient cards were identified with short-term affective behavioral responses (TABR); during this survey of clinical data on the presence of formed BMD in this group which was not revealed, they were provided with psychocorrectional assistance by psychologists at the place of service. (c) Three hundred fifteen people (19.8%)—they were identified with adaptation disorders (RA) and PTSD; in this regard therapy and medical and psychological rehabilitation were carried out.

Three hundred eleven combatants were identified as having different TABR, which were recorded in the outpatient records of combatants by psychiatrists or neurologists during the 6-year period preceding our study (Group 1). These states occurred in the form of short-term emotional-maladaptive states and behavioral disorders and belonged to the pre-painful level (305 people). In Group 2 clinically formed BMD were revealed: AD was observed in 166 people (54.4%), among them are short-term depressive reaction (F 43.20)—35 (21.1%), prolonged depressive reaction (F 43.21)—31 (18.6%), mixed anxiety and depressive reaction (F 43.22)—35 (21.1%), violations of other emotions (F 43.23)—21 (12.6%), with prevalence of behavior disorders (F 43.24)—34 (20.5%), and mixed disorder of emotions and behavior (F 43.25)—10 (6.1%). Clinically designed PTSD was diagnosed in 139 people (45.6%) including anxiety type—36 (25.9%), explosive—33 (23.9%), somatoform—38 (27.6%), and conversion—31 (22.6%).

Our data confirm the studies of many authors who note the high prevalence of BMD among combatants around the world (especially in recent decades), which is associated with the extreme nature of service and participation in the settlement of ethnic conflicts [12, 17].

The combatants from the AD had emotional disorders in the form of anxiety and depression, periodically arising dysphoria of different severities depending on the clinical variant of the AD. All combatants registered a violation of interpersonal communication with a pronounced irritability, hot temper, and distrust of others.

Dreams of combat content in all combatants with PTSD presented painful scenes with a sense of threat to life ("could not defend"; "shot, but the bullets flew by"; "the corpses of the dead came to life"); dreams were accompanied by fear and vegetative symptoms (heartbeat, sweating). Depression, oppressive tension that is not a characteristic of earlier, increased sensitivity to everyday stimuli (loud sounds, the smell of gunpowder, gasoline), alertness, suspicion, and "over vigilance" were noted. There was a fear of open spaces with a sense of threat from the outside (squares, markets, and lawns were associated with "stretch marks," fear of undermining, unfinished buildings with the threat of sniper fire, death, pits on construction sites with "graves," and mass death of people).

Clinical manifestations of PTSD differed depending on the course of the disease. In combatants with an alarming type of PTSD, the structure of the disease was dominated by the symptoms of the neurotic circle: unmotivated anxiety, frequent mood changes, sleep disorders (difficulty in falling asleep, early awakenings, lack of a sense of rest after a night's sleep), lethargy, weakness, and "heaviness in the head."

In persons with an explosive type of PTSD, pronounced irritability and discontent were observed. They were characterized by resentment, vindictiveness, hostility to others, a tendency to solve everyday problems with the help of physical force, alertness, suspicion, vulnerability, and negativity. On the background of the overall tension, reducing the adaptive capacity of the neurotic tendency to impulsive reactions traced the difficulty in volitional control of negative emotions in everyday life; various forms of maladaptive behavior, such as excessive alcohol consumption and episodic use of psychoactive substances (PAS), were observed.

The structure of somatoform-type PTSD was dominated by pain in the region of the heart, in the course of the gastrointestinal tract. There was a pronounced hypochondriac fixation on these symptoms and an alarming expectation of their amplification, which forced patients to contact general practitioners, at the same time, periodically stated functional cardio-pathologies, dizziness, neuralgia, sleep disorders, headaches, nausea, vomiting, urological manifestations, and sexual dysfunction.

In combatants with a conversion type of PTSD in the clinic, the symptoms of increasing excitement with a lack of criticality to the disease prevailed, acute demonstrative reactions to external stimuli associated with the main traumatic factor, unmotivated initiative, increased chatter, inflated self-esteem, and the search for "perpetrators of the tragedy" with the desire for revenge. There were episodes of affective narrowing of consciousness with bouts of rage, physical aggression, and lack of guilt.

Analysis of clinical symptoms in TABR and BMD combatants showed that PTSD symptoms, such as reliving traumatic events and nightmares, were observed in both groups of combatants but were significantly more frequent in Group 2. "Flashback" symptoms with pronounced psychosomatic manifestations in the form of tachycardia, sweating, and increased blood pressure with repeated trauma are recorded in both groups but most often in combatants with BMD. Hallucinations when falling asleep were only observed in individuals of Group 2. Dissociative manifestations to trigger the incentives in the structure of symptom re-experiencing the traumatic event are significantly more prevalent in individuals with the TABR in history.

Phobic reactions to trigger stimuli were found in groups with approximately the same frequency. Avoidance of thoughts, feelings, and people (everything that reminded about the injury) was revealed in both groups of respondents, but the frequency is significantly higher in persons with BMD (**Table 1**).

It should be noted that combatants with TABR were significantly more likely to have psychogenic amnesia in the structure of the avoidance symptom than those with BDM.

Symptoms		TABR		BMD		P
		n = 311	%	n = 305	%	
At the moment of threat	Amnesia	0	0	1	0,3	0.345
	Fear	0	0	1	0.3	0.456
	Disorganization of behavior	5	1.6	6	1.9	0.367
	Narrowing of consciousness	0	0	6	1.9	0.458
Repeated experiences	"Flashback" symptoms	79	25.4	195	63,9	<0.001
	Nightmares	58	18.6	136	44,6	<0.001
	Hallucinations when falling asleep	0	0	10	3.3	465
	Phobic reactions on the trigger incentives	3	0.9	4	1.3	0.478
	Dissociative symptoms on the trigger incentives	12	3.9	6	1.9	<0.05
Avoidance	Thoughts, feelings	11	3.5	38	12.5	< 0.05
	Human action	69	22.9	143	46.8	<0.001
	Psychogenic fugue	12	3.9	4	1.3	< 0.05
	Reduced interest in previously Significant events	9	2.9	92	30.2	<0,001
	Sense of detachment, isolation	7	2.3	29	9.5	< 0.05
	The decrease in the level of Emotional response	34	10.9	89	29.2	<0.001
	The feeling of lack of perspective	0	0	12	3.9	0.478
Excitations	Sleep disturbance	89	28.6	198	64.9	< 0.05
	Irritability	78	25.1	264	86.5	< 0.05
	Temper	96	30.9	214	70.1	<0.001
	Violations of concentration of Attention	32	10.2	139	45.6	<0.001
Signs of social and labor maladjustment		9	2.9	45	14.6	<0.001

Note: P is calculated using Pearson's χ^2, and intergroup differences were significant at $p < 0.05$.

Table 1.
Frequency of post-traumatic symptoms and stress disorders in combatants with BMD and TABR (%).

Symptoms of emotional deficits with social introversion, such as a decrease in interest in previously significant events, a sense of detachment and isolation, and a decrease in the level of emotional response were found in both groups of respondents but were significantly more often present in people with BDM. A sense of lack of perspective was present in individuals with only clinically formed BDM (**Table 1**).

In the combatant with TABR, clinical symptoms included maladaptive emotional and behavioral responses with symptoms characteristic of PTSD, but their duration and severity were significantly shorter and did not fit into the clinical criteria of the disease. In persons from the group with PPR, clinical symptoms were more pronounced, long-lasting, and polymorphic.

3. Features of therapy and rehabilitation of borderline mental disorders in combatants

Active and timely diagnosis of adverse mental health conditions in combatants, rehabilitation, and therapeutic measures is an urgent task of the departmental health [15].

Many researchers noted the importance of developing new approaches to the treatment and rehabilitation of combatants with BMD. Inconsistency in psychodiagnostic approaches and terminology often leads to disagreements of specialists and is an obstacle to the modern provision of the necessary complex medical and psychological care.

Rehabilitation is a complex of consistently held measures of medical, social, psychological, and pedagogical nature, aimed at the restoration of the individual to the level of her social activity.

An important aspect of the success of BMD therapy is a personality-oriented approach that takes into account premorbid personality characteristics [7]. Combatants with harmonious traits, BMD treatment, and social readaptation are more successful in the near and in the remote period after participation in the war.

Psychotherapists identify the main directions of psychotherapy of combatants with combat mental trauma: restoration of a sense of value of life, control over their emotions, and restoration of destroyed social positive attitudes [12]. At the same time, the proposed techniques of work, long-term enough that in real conditions of service with existing employees is almost impossible to implement.

At an early stage, as the practice of military conflicts in Afghanistan, the Persian Gulf, Vietnam, shows, it is advisable to carefully identify combatants who have received battle mental injuries and to maintain confidentiality, as the mechanism of "psychiatric stigma" is included. "Fatigue after a fight" in most cases is transformed into PTSD, which is a natural reaction of a person who finds himself in a war.

O. Yurkovsky fully described the stages and types of rehabilitation treatment of combatants with BMD, which include a set of medical, psychological, and social measures in inpatient and outpatient settings. The rehabilitation of patients with PTSD in the form of organization of the school, the basic principles of which are: balance, adaptability, and prevention; stages and continuity; complexity; and the concept of psychosocial rehabilitation of veterans of the war in Afghanistan, including three stages, is described: allocation of the main streams of combatants; conducting the main rehabilitation course (using special assistance centers); and supporting medical, psychological, and social methods [20].

Development of the organization of necessary assistance to combatants should be based on a multi-professional, integrated approach with brigade methods and involvement of psychiatrists, psychotherapists, clinical psychologists, and drug addicts (in connection with the epidemic of drug use in the world and in Russia in particular). The most significant strategic miscalculation of the rehabilitation service creation is that the foundation on which the service is built is not defined [18].

Many experts in the field of mental health noted that the rehabilitation and therapy of veterans of combat operations are not sufficient; in this regard, they have the most pronounced risk of BMD and deviant behavior, which leads to a decrease in professional reliability and social functioning in general [11, 19].

S. Litvintsev notes that the treatment of persons with PTSD is advisable to produce in specialized departments and centers; the system of which in our country has not yet been established [9].

The sequence and complexity of rehabilitation treatment are dictated by the need to resocialize combatants to reduce the negative psychosocial consequences in the modern society [7, 13].

When treating and rehabilitating combatants with PTSD, it is important to balance clinical and social approaches and motivate patients to recover quickly.

In literature there are conflicting data on the evaluation of the effectiveness of therapy and rehabilitation of participants in hostilities. The analysis of the long-term results of rehabilitation measures conducted by O. Yurkovsky [20] showed that 88.5% of patients were successfully adapted and the effectiveness of treatment remained during the year. The effectiveness of therapy and rehabilitation depends on the timeliness of treatment, favorable premorbid, social support, and the absence of concomitant somatic diseases [8].

Rehabilitation of persons with combat PTSD is a complex problem requiring improvement of organizational approaches and development of programs with the participation of various specialists involved in mental health.

The use of psychopharmacotherapy in the treatment of BMD in combatants allows to stop psychopathological symptoms in the early stages, to increase the effectiveness of crisis psychotherapy, to reduce anxiety and aggression, to neutralize negative emotional reactions, and to improve interpersonal communication and social interaction.

The choice of methods of medical treatment of BMD in combatants is based on clinical symptoms and is prescribed taking into account the main psychopathological syndromes and clinical forms in accordance with the standards of psychiatric care.

With the predominance of depressive symptoms in the picture of BMD, it is advisable to use antidepressants (selective serotonin reuptake inhibitors and tricyclic antidepressants).

In the case of the presence of PTSD and AD structure of alarming symptoms with sleep disorders, short course of explosive prescribe benzodiazepine tranquilizers and/or small neuroleptics.

In conversion disorders, behavior correctors are mainly used. Antidepressants are not used due to the fact that they increase the dissociative symptoms.

In the case of an explosive version of PTSD and AD, behavioral disorders are corrected with drugs with predominantly sedative effect; in some cases, a good effect is observed when taking lithium drugs due to stabilization of the emotional state.

In the treatment of short-term depressive reactions caused by AD and PTSD with symptoms of anxiety and depression, selective serotonin reuptake inhibitors are most often used.

A good effect in the treatment of PPR, in the structure of which is dominated by anxiety and hypochondriac symptoms, as well as insomnia is noted when using benzodiazepine tranquilizers in the course 2–3 weeks, with gradual abolition.

In combatants due to the negative impact of stresses of official activity after the execution of operational tasks in special conditions, often there are situational-due affective reactions, which are accompanied by anxiety and anxiety-phobic symptoms, which require the use of drugs with anxiolytic action. Their advantage is the absence of addiction and withdrawal syndrome, as well as a minimum number of side effects.

In addition to drug therapy, combatants with BMD are provided with psychotherapy to respond to negative feelings and change attitudes to traumatic events. The main difficulty is the establishment of trusting contact, which is associated with the characteristics of patients that expressed distrust of the environment.

When conducting psychotherapy at the initial stage of medical rehabilitation, the presence of "combatant accentuation," in the structure of which there is a formed distrust, unwillingness to seek help, skepticism, difficulties in interpersonal communication, and increased irritability and temper. These features often lead to conflicts with medical staff and psychologists. In combatants with PTSD, preference is given to individual forms of psychotherapy, especially at the stationary stage, since collective and group psychotherapy in the stage of acute clinical symptoms causes protest reactions in some people with BMD in the form of explosive outbreaks and dissociative symptoms.

The establishment of empathic, trusting relationships between the patient and the psychotherapist is a critical therapeutic factor necessary for the effectiveness of therapy. When building communication in the process of psychotherapeutic treatment, it is necessary to take into account the personal characteristics of patients [3].

Psychotherapy with combatants is aimed at:

* Formation of motivation for treatment and overcoming of the stigmatized attitude to the treatment process.
* Combatant study of their psychological and personal characteristics.
  • Correction of response patterns in civilian life.
* Formation of adaptive behavior skills in the service and at home.
  • Training in the techniques of psychical self-regulation and increase of their psychological capabilities for gaining control of emotional reactions.

At the initial stage of rehabilitation, it is advisable to conduct individual rational psychotherapy with all combatants—for the interpretation of the nature and causes of traumatic stress through logical re-persuasion, the formation of motivation for psychotherapeutic treatment, and overcoming the stigmatized attitude to psychotherapeutic assistance. The means of psychological influence are persuasion, explanation, and distraction. The main purpose of this psychotherapeutic method is to study the patient's personality, evaluation, and correction of inadequate emotional and behavioral stereotypes of the patient, which determine the violation of his psychological and social functioning.

The use of art therapy contributes to the additional diagnosis of personal problems, affective disorders, further de-actualization of traumatic events, the expansion of adaptive reserves, self-esteem, and mood correction. The plot should be connected with the peculiarities of the combatants' attitude, feelings, and experiences reflecting the stressful effects. The therapy is conducted individually and effective combatants as with adjustment disorder, and PTSD. Painting and drawing techniques are used with various materials (gouache, pencil, oil, watercolor, artistic coal). Depending on the material chosen by the combatant, the duration of the session is from 30 minutes to 1.5 hours, and the number of sessions per course of therapy is from 3 to 10 times.

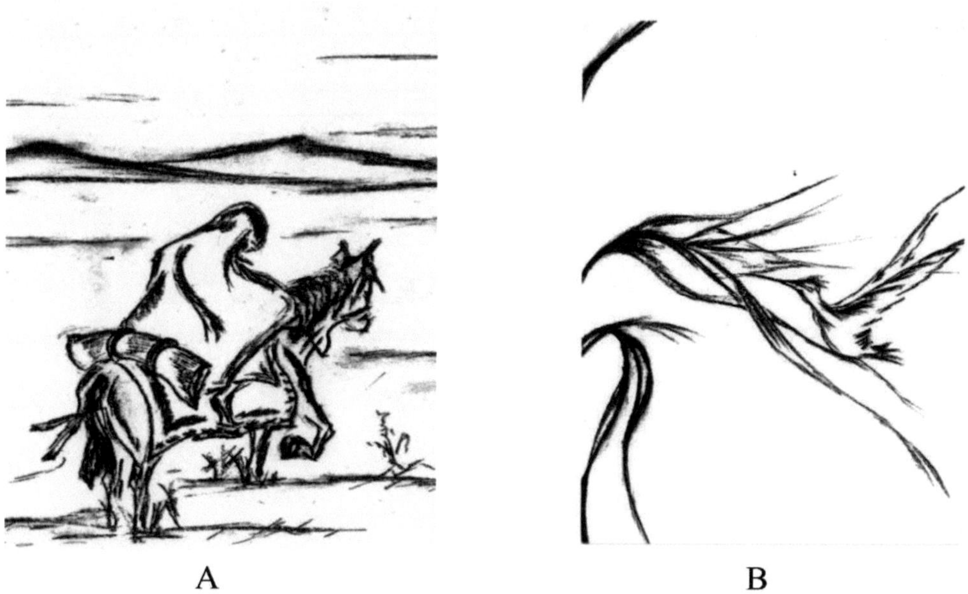

Figure 1.
(A) Combatant K—Before treatment. Diagnosis: PTSD, dysphoric type. (B) Combatant K—In a month of therapy.

As an example, illustrating the theoretical material, we present the work of two combatants diagnosed with PTSD. A work of art is made with charcoal.

In the examination of combatant K, 27 years old, after returning from the NCR, he was found to have pronounced explosive and dysphoric symptoms, the violation of communicative processes, social isolation, pessimism, and a diagnosis of PTSD, dysphoric type (a plot—"a lone rider," **Figure 1A**).

After the medical and psychological rehabilitation, improvement of the emotional background and reduction of the main psychopathological manifestations were noted (a plot —"nest," **Figure 1B**).

During the examination of combatant M. after returning from the NCR (a plot—"warrior," **Figure 2A**), there was a pronounced aggressive-dysphoric mood, violation of interpersonal communication skills, negativity, and "defensive position." After the medical and psychological rehabilitation, the stability of the emotional background, balance, and reducing anxiety and aggression were noted (a plot—"sea, calm," **Figure 2B**).

In the works of the combatant K, 27 years old, diagnosed with PTSD, an alarming type, there was also a positive dynamics of mental state. A work of art is made with charcoal. After returning from the NCR (a plot—"a wolf howls at the moon"), expressed anxiety and depression symptoms, a violation of communication processes, social isolation, and pessimism were noted (**Figure 3A**). After the medical and psychological rehabilitation (a plot—"winter landscape"), the stability of the emotional background, balance, and lack of anxiety and depression on the background of introversion were noted (**Figure 3B**).

The leading method in working with combatants is family psychotherapy, aimed at restoring family values and interpersonal relations in the family. The attention of the immediate environment is focused on the need to provide psychological assistance and family support to the combatants; it is explained that the return to peaceful life may be accompanied by difficulties. Family members are given a description of the combatant's behavior, the problems that have arisen after combat stress are reported to be of a nonpermanent nature, and the family can help to deal with them.

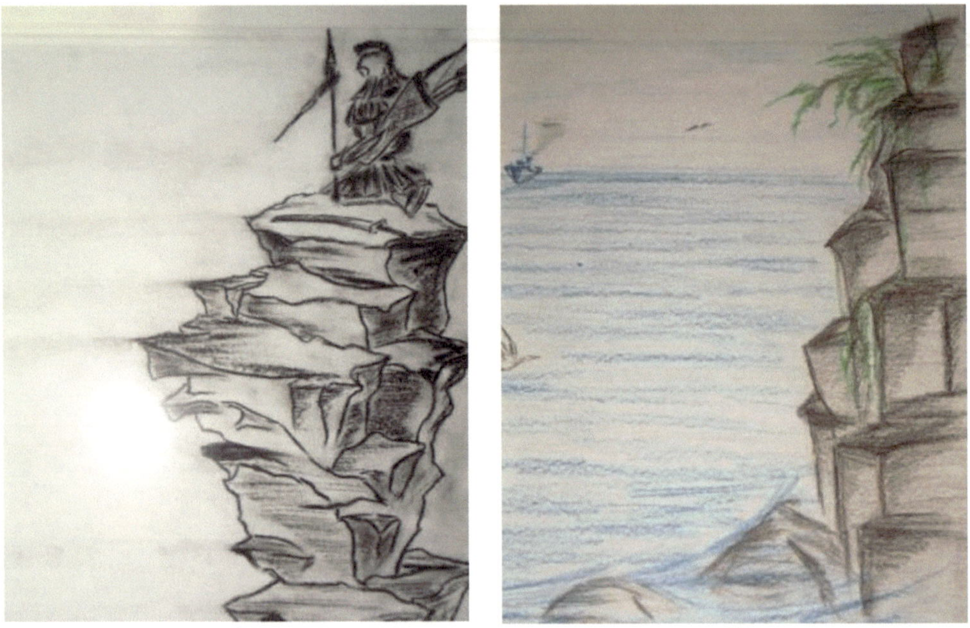

A B

Figure 2.
(A) Combatant M—Before treatment. Diagnosis: PTSD. (B) Combatant M—in a month of therapy.

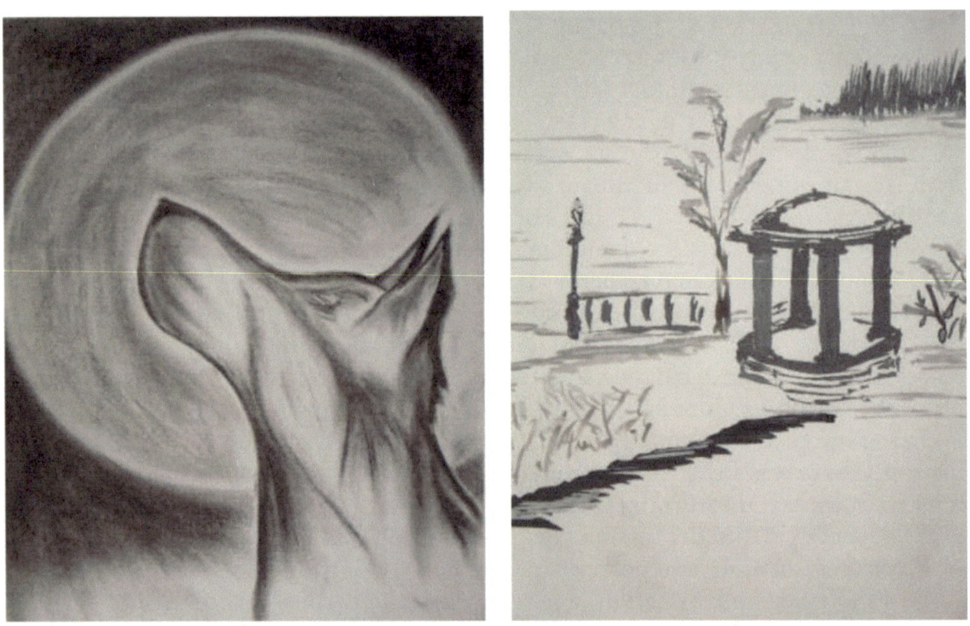

A B

Figure 3.
(A) Combatant K—Before treatment. Diagnosis: PTSD. (B) Combatant K—in a month of therapy.

Our data in the study of mental morbidity among combatants significantly differ from the studies of O. Shevtsova and V. Kokhanova, who revealed that the background of the increase in the number of BMD, dismissal among the military who underwent BND, is 61.4% due to clinical resistance to therapy and the presence of psychosocial consequences [19]. Similar data are noted in the works of

D. Svechnikov and co-authors, who show that neurotic disorders in military personnel are the leading pathology for defense agencies, leading to early dismissal and extremely negative impact on the combat effectiveness of the army [11].

According to our data, the timely provision of professional assistance to combatants with the BMD not only does not lead to dismissal but also is not an obstacle to professional growth. In the process of rehabilitation of combatants with BMD, there is a positive trend: a month after the start of therapy in persons with RA is 83.3% and PTSD in 67.4% of cases; during the year 93.1 and 89.9% and in 4 years 98.9 and 96.6%, respectively. V. Shamrey noted that the identified violations in the combatants rarely led to a serious violation of social adaptation but felt sick as hindering the possibility of adequate realization of their personal potential; they did not associate them with the disease, regarded them as "growing up" [17].

Thus, early detection of BMD and pre-pain conditions in combatants with appropriate poly-professional therapy leads to positive results, contributing not only to the preservation of mental health but also to further career growth.

Author details

Andrey Soloviev[1]*, Elena Ichitovkina[2] and Marina Zlokazova[2]

1 Northern State Medical University, Arkhangelsk, Russia

2 Kirov State Medical University, Kirov, Russia

*Address all correspondence to: asoloviev1@yandex.ru

References

[1] Alexandrovsky Yu. Psychogeny in extreme conditions/Yu.Alexandrovsky, O.Lobastov, L.Spivak. - Moscow: Medicine, 1991. 96 p

[2] Aksenov M. Post-traumatic stress disorder in some types of professional activity: problem / M.Aksenov, N.Reginas V.Petrov // Bulletin of the Tomsk State Pedagogical University. - 2014. - № 5 (146) P. 117-122

[3] Boyko E. Quality of life of combatants with chronic PTSD and its Dynamics (Pembroke, Ont.) as the result of Rehabilitation measures / E.Boyko, A.Pogosov, Yu.Sochivko // Siberian Bulletin of Psychiatry and Narcology. 2012. № 1. P. 19-22

[4] Voloshin V. Clinical typology of post-traumatic stress disorders and issues of differentiated psychopharmacotherapy / V.Voloshin // psychiatry and Psycho-Pharmacotherapy 2001. Vol. 3, № 4. P. 125-132

[5] Gracheva L. Socio-psychological adaptation and psychosomatic disorders in individuals with combat stress History/L.Gracheva, V.Sergeev// Scientific Notes State Medical University named after I.P.Pavlov. - 2013. Vol. XX, № 4. P. 41-44

[6] Epanchintseva E. Clinical structure of mental disorders in participants of local armed conflicts in the distant post-boom period / E.Epanchintseva, T.Kazennych, V.Lebedev, N.Bokhan // advances in modern Natural Science. - 2015. № 1-5. P. 760-764

[7] Ichitovkina E. Systematic monitoring of Mental Health of the combatants – police officers / E.Ichetovkina, M.Zlokazova, A.Soloviev Arkhangelsk: Publishing House of The Northern State Medical University, 2017. 205 p

[8] Ichetovkina E. Predicting the emergence of prenosological mental disorders in combatants / E.Ichitovkina, M.Zlokazova, A.Soloviev, O.Kharkova, G.Shutko // Human Ecology. 2016. No. 10. P. 47-50

[9] Litvintsev S. Combat trauma: A guide for physicians / V.Litvintsev, E.Snetkov, A.Reznik. – Moscow: JSC Publishing House "Medicine", 2005. 345 p

[10] Marchenko A. Problematic issues of diagnosis and pathomorphism of neurotic disorders among military Personnel / A.Marchenko, V.Shamrey, V.Nechiporenko, I.Rudoy, A.Krasnov, O.Pushkina // DoctorRu. 2012. № 5 (73). P. 61-66

[11] Svechnikov D. Objective diagnosis of adjustment disorder in military / D.Svechnikov, N.Baurova, T.Ushakova, E.Kurasov // El Médico-Biological and Socio-Psychological Problems in Emergency Situations - 2014. № 4. P. 40-44

[12] Snedkov V. Medical and psychological consequences of battle mental Trauma: clinical, dynamic and therapeutic and Rehabilitation aspects / V.Snedkov, S.Litvintsev, V.Nechiporenko, V.Lytkin / / Modern Psychiatry. 2008. № 3. P. 21-25

[13] Soloviev A. Dynamics of formation of psychic disorders of combatants and pensioners of the Ministry of Internal Affairs / A.Soloviev, A.Shutov, M.Zlokazova, E.Ichitovkina /// Advances in Gerantology. - 2017, T.30. No. 6. P. 912-916

[14] Sukisyan S. Post-traumatic stress disorder among former combatants from functional to organic / S.Sukiasyan, M.Tadevosyan / Psychiatry. 2011. № 1 (49). P. 59-69

[15] Phastoutov G. Expert Criteria for the Application of Article 22 of the Criminal Code of the Russian Federation in Individuals with Atypical Variants of PTSD / G.Phastoutov, E.Zaitsev // Psychiatry in the Stage of Reforms: Problems and Prospects. XVI Congress of Psychiatrists of Russia Kazan, 2015. pp. 866-867

[16] Phisun A. Ways of prevention of addictive disorders in the army / a.Phisun, V.Shamrey, A.Marchenko, A.Semenchenko, A.Pastushenkov // Military Medical Journal. 2013. Vol. 334, No. 9. P. 4-10

[17] Shamrey V. Residual deficitary status in disorders of neurotic Spectrum V.Shamrey, A.Marchenko, E.Abritalin, A.Krasnov, A.Goncharenko // Social and Clinical Psychiatry. 2013. Vol. 23, № 4. P. 14-18

[18] Shevchenko N. Temperament as a Characteristic of the Main Properties of the Nervous System of Employees of the Federal Fire Service / N.Shevchenko T.Makarova // Medico-Biological and Socio-Psychological Problems in Emergency Situations. Vol. 1. 2015 pp. 115-119

[19] Shevtsova O. The features of the initial changes in mental health status from the military intelligence agencies of Russia / O.Shevtsova, V.Kokhanov // Emergency Medicine. 2010. № 1. P. 30-33

[20] Yurkovsky *O. Complex* system of rehabilitation of patients with post-stress disorders/O.Yurkovsky, Yu.Zamotaev. - Moscow: Medicine, 2006. 233 p

Chapter 6

Prevalence and Treatment of Anxiety Disorders Comorbidities in a Clinical Romanian Sample of Children and Adolescents with Psychiatric Disorders

Elena Predescu, Anna Boglarka Asztalos and Roxana Șipoș

Abstract

The prevalence of anxiety disorders is known to be increasing among children and adolescents and often co-exist with another psychiatric disorder. There is some evidence that anxiety disorders in nonwestern countries have the same comorbidity patterns as in other world regions and may have similar predictors including age and gender. However, more evidence from different countries is needed. The major goal of the study was to evaluate the prevalence of anxiety disorders in a clinical setting and to describe the comorbidity patterns and predictors. We conducted a retrospective study on the admitted patients in the Clinic of Pediatric Psychiatry from Cluj-Napoca, Romania, between January 2017 and December 2017. A clinical sample of 2471 patients aged between 3 and 18 years with psychiatric disorders, assessed and/or treated in the clinic, was included into the study. About 9.88% patients (N = 244) of the clinical sample were diagnosed with an anxiety disorder as a primary diagnosis. About 79.5% of the selected sample had a comorbid disorder and 34.4% had an anxiety or mood comorbidity. Preference in treatment was nonpharmachological and, according to the degree of severity, SSRI medication. Our results underline the significant prevalence of anxiety disorders and the high rate of comorbidities.

Keywords: anxiety disorders, prevalence, comorbidities, children and adolescents, pharmacological treatment

1. Introduction

1.1 Diagnostic systems

Anxiety disorders (ADs) are one of the most important conditions in child and adolescent psychiatry with a heterogeneous spectrum of clinical manifestations and variable levels of severity. ADs are commonly found at all levels of mental health services and involve the use of large resources for the appropriate assessment and therapeutic approach.

Anxiety disorders (ADs) are classified in *DSM-5* (APA) [1] or *ICD-10* (WHO) [2] diagnostic systems. Although developmental pathway features or a variety of other factors can significantly influence clinical presentation, both classification systems describe common clinical features for AD [3] and use roughly the same diagnosis criteria for children and adolescents as compared to adults. *ICD-10*, in contrast to *DSM-5*, uses several separate diagnostic codes for children. The new proposed disorder categories in *ICD-11* are largely the same as those in the equivalent section of *DSM-5* and recognize that the same disorders occur across the life span with developmentally distinct presentations [4]. Therefore, diagnoses in *ICD* are made based on essential features, with the expectation that the clinicians will use their clinical judgment on exact symptom counts and duration in a manner that is consistent with the diagnostic guidance provided [5]. Although this descriptive diagnosis criteria facilitated the development of diagnostic instruments for AD assessment [6–10], clinicians should be aware of their limitations, particularly related to developmental issues in obtaining self-reports from children and adolescents [11]. Due to these considerations, the core diagnostic criteria might present differently in the young, requiring special assessment strategies.

1.2 Prevalence

Mental disorders affect a significant number of children and adolescents worldwide [12]. Among the children and adolescent psychiatric disorders, ADs are a representative category. Prevalence rates reported in studies are varying considerably sometimes, depending on the sample, assessment methods, the assessed period, or study design, between 6.5 [12] and 8.3% [13] and up to 27% [14]. In a meta-analysis of multiple data sets, Costello et al. have found the prevalence of 10.2% for any AD, 5.4% for specific phobia (SPEC), 3.6% for social phobia (SOC), 2.6% for separation anxiety disorder (SAD), 1.7% for generalized anxiety disorder (GAD), and 0.8% for panic disorder (PD) [15]. In the National Comorbidity Survey Replication and Adolescent Supplement, Kessler et al. reported a lifetime prevalence of any anxiety disorders of 32.4%, for the ages of 3–17 [16]. Spence et al.'s results are slightly different, with reported prevalence rates of 2.3% for social phobia (SOC), 4.3% for separation anxiety (SAD), and 2.2% for generalized anxiety disorder (GAD) [17]. Previous studies reported similar prevalence rates in diverse cultures [18–20].

In terms of onset age, Merikangas et al. found a prevalence of 31.4% for the age group of 13–14 years, 32.1% for the age group of 15–16 years, and 32.3% for the age group of 17–18 years, with particularly high rates of specific phobia (SPEC) [13]. Generalized anxiety disorder and social anxiety disorder are among the most common AD in youth [21]. Panic disorder is rare and occurs in adolescents rather than in young children [15, 21]. Findings from different studies have demonstrated that, in the general population, anxiety symptoms first decrease during early adolescence and subsequently increase from middle to late adolescence [22]. Separation anxiety disorder and specific phobias tend to emerge and predominate during childhood, whereas the initial onset of generalized anxiety disorder, panic disorder, and social anxiety disorder most often occurs during adolescence [16, 23].

The literature describes the theory on distinct latent developmental trajectories for different anxiety disorder symptoms, emphasizing the importance of examining separate anxiety dimensions rather than considering anxiety as a general construct. For example, girls were significantly more likely than boys to be in numerous latent generalized anxiety disorder symptom trajectory classes, including those distinguished by very high initial symptoms that decrease rapidly, high initial symptoms that decrease less markedly over time, and moderate initial symptoms that decrease slightly over time [24]. The results from Crocetti et al.'s study regarding latent growth trajectory classes found that adolescent population was best typified by a low-anxiety class, characterized by a low initial anxiety level that decreased over time and a high-anxiety class characterized by a higher initial anxiety level that increased over time [25]. In a 5-year study of Dutch, youth aged between 10 and 12 years at baseline, generalized anxiety disorder, panic disorder, and social anxiety disorder symptoms slightly decreased and then leveled off from early to middle adolescence, followed by a slight increase in generalized anxiety disorder and social anxiety disorder symptoms during middle adolescence and in panic disorder symptoms during late adolescence [22, 26]. Similar results have been reported by recent studies [24, 27].

There are mixed data regarding the differential gender prevalence rates of anxiety. Similar to gender ratio for adults, girls tend to have more of all subtypes of anxiety disorders, but there is no significant difference between boys and girls in the mean age at onset of anxiety [28]. Some studies showed that girls have a higher risk to develop AD [13, 16], are more affected [13, 24], and report higher cross-sectional anxiety symptom levels [29–31], and these differences remain stable during adolescence [20].

1.3 Comorbidities

Generally, in child and adolescent psychiatry, the comorbidities are the rule, and anxiety disorders fit into this pattern. In the clinical practice, AD comorbidities in internalization symptom area are commonly identified and closely monitored compared with the externalization symptoms. However, there are very few papers focused on the comorbidity between specific anxiety disorders and other psychiatric diagnoses.

Comorbidity occurs frequently, both within the anxiety disorders and also with other psychiatric disorders. At least one third of the children and adolescents diagnosed with anxiety disorders meet the criteria for two or more anxiety disorders [32]. Children with a primary anxiety disorder were significantly more likely to be diagnosed with separation anxiety disorder than adolescents. Adolescents with a primary anxiety disorder received more frequently a primary diagnosis of social anxiety disorder, mood disorders, and irregular school attendance [33]. Anxiety disorders are associated with all the other major classes of disorders, including mood disorders, disruptive behaviors, ADHD, eating disorders, and substance use disorders [19, 28, 34–36]. Merikangas et al. reported in their national survey among adolescents aged 13–18 years that the anxiety disorders were the most common condition (31.9%), with approximately 40% of those with one class of disorder also meeting criteria for another class of lifetime disorder [13]. Costello et al. found that comorbidity with other psychiatric disorders was common, ranging from 53% of the generalized anxiety disorder cases to 100% of specific phobia cases. The most common type of comorbidity with non-anxiety disorders was with depression [15, 20, 37, 38]. Adolescents with high levels of depressive symptoms experienced less significant decline over time in symptoms of physical, social, and separation anxiety [30]. The Oregon Adolescent Depression Study, looking at lifetime diagnoses, revealed that depression was significantly associated with each of the anxiety disorders except obsessive-compulsive disorder. Other lifetime associations found were ADHD with specific phobia and bipolar disorder with separation anxiety in males [39]. In preschool children, Sterba et al. used confirmatory factor analysis to show that the best-fitting model for the emotional disorders had three factors (social phobia, separation anxiety, and a factor that combined GAD and depression) with significant correlations between these three factors and conduct disorder, oppositional disorder, and

ADHD [40–42]. Social, separation, and generalized anxiety disorders in young people are relatively common and with a high level of comorbidity. All three ADs have a relatively high level of comorbidity with depression and a moderate degree of comorbidity with ADHD [17].

The major goal of the present study was to assess the prevalence of anxiety disorders among children and adolescents in a clinical setting and to describe the comorbidity and pharmacological treatment patterns.

2. Method

2.1 Participant selection

We conducted a retrospective study on the admitted patients in the Clinic of Pediatric Psychiatry from Cluj-Napoca, Romania, between January and December 2017. A clinical sample of 2471 patients aged between 3 and 18 years, with different psychiatric disorders, assessed and/or treated in the clinic, was included in the study. 9.88% (N = 244) of the clinical sample were children and adolescents diagnosed with an anxiety disorder via the 10th revision of the *International Statistical Classification of Diseases and Related Health Problems (ICD 10)*-based clinical interviews. Participants were grouped according to the "primary" diagnosis, the primary diagnosis referring to the severity of current diagnoses and not the order of onset (the reason for admission). In accordance with the removal of OCD and PTSD from the broad anxiety disorders category in *DSM-5* (American Psychiatric Association, 2013), the patients with a primary diagnosis of OCD and PTSD were excluded from this study.

We included in the study: boys or girls aged 3–18 with a diagnosis of anxiety disorders (agoraphobia; social phobias; specific phobias; other/unspecified phobic anxiety disorders; panic disorder; generalized anxiety disorder; mixed anxiety and depressive disorder; other mixed, specified, or unspecified anxiety disorders; separation anxiety disorder of childhood; social anxiety disorder of childhood), according to *ICD-10* international diagnosis criteria, admitted for assessment or treatment; agreement (children/adolescent and caregiver) to participate after the purpose and protocol of the study was explained. We excluded from the study: children and adolescents admitted with other diagnosis than anxiety disorders and the patients receiving services in outpatient settings.

Data were collected from the patients' medical records (sociodemographic, clinical evaluations, and treatment recommendations). From the total of the 2471 patients selected, 244 children and adolescents were diagnosed with a type of anxiety disorder as a primary diagnosis. The patients come from all the countries and are diverse in terms of socioeconomic status. The mean age of participants was 12.75 (SD = 3.90), their age ranging from 3 to 18 years. All the participants were Caucasian. Data were used ensuring the privacy and subject's identity protection.

2.2 Statistical analysis

The Statistical Program for Social Sciences (SPSS) v. 17 was used for data analysis. To describe and assess the selected population, we used univariate statistical analysis (mean, standard deviation, frequencies). Pearson chi-square test was used to verify the association among categorical variables, and t-test was used to compare the mean age. The level of significance was set at 5%, and a confidence interval (CI) of 95% was used in all tests.

2.3 Results

Two hundred forty-four patients with a primary diagnosis of anxiety disorder were included in the study of which 130 (53.3%) were males and 114 (46.7%) were females. The boy-girl ratio was 1.14:1. The mean age of boys and girls differs significantly (mean (SD) boys = 12.02 (4.08), girls = 13.60 (3.52), t = −3.24, p = 0.001).

2.3.1 Primary disorder prevalence

We analized the prevalence data for all anxiety disorder diagnosis of the patients included in the study, with current ICD 10 principal diagnosis are presented. As seen in **Table 1**, the most commonly occurring diagnosis were generalized anxiety disorder (GAD) 35.7% of the sample, social phobias (SOC) 12.3%, mixed anxiety and depressive (MAD) disorder 11.5%, other specified anxiety disorders (OSA) 9%, and separation anxiety disorder (SAD) of childhood 8.6%. The other anxiety disorders were less represented in our sample: specific phobias (SPEC) 6.1%, other phobic anxiety disorders (NOS) 4.9%, anxiety disorder, unspecified (ADU) 3.7%, panic disorder (PD) 3.3%, other mixed anxiety disorders (OMAD) 1.6%, phobic anxiety disorder, unspecified (UNS) 0.8%, and social anxiety disorder of childhood (SADC) 0.8%. About 20.5% of the sample (N = 50) had only 1 diagnosis at admission, 46.7% (N = 114) had 2 diagnoses, and 32.8% (N = 80) had 3 or more clinical diagnoses. Comorbidity is defined as having two or more co-occurring current diagnoses. **Table 1** presents the prevalence of the additional diagnosis for the participants grouped by the principal diagnosis. 34.4% of the participants had a diagnosis of anxiety or depressive disorder in addition to their principal anxiety disorder diagnosis. The other frequent comorbidities were attention deficit hyperactivity disorder (ADHD) (28.7%) and autism spectrum disorder (ASD) (8.6%).

2.3.2 Age and gender

The participants were divided into two groups by age: children (N = 88; 3–11 years of age) and adolescents (N = 156; 12–18 years of age). Among participants who met diagnostic criteria for the targeted anxiety disorders (N = 244), adolescents were significantly more likely to receive a principal diagnosis of GAD than children (39.7 vs. 28.4%, chi-square = 13.11, p < 0.001) or MAD (13.5 vs. 8%, chi-square = 9.33, p = 0.02). The prevalences of generalized anxiety disorder (GAD) and mixed anxiety and depressive (MAD) disorder were found higher in adolescents than in children (**Table 1**), but with a higher prevalence in adolescent girls, the proportion of boys diagnosed with GAD and MAD being relatively stable with age. Children were more likely to receive a principal diagnosis of SPEC than adolescents (11.4 vs. 3.2%, chi-square = 3.75, p = 0.05). For specific phobias (SPEC), the prevalence was higher in children than in adolescents, but while the proportion of boys remained relatively stable, the diagnosis wasn't present in adolescent girls.

No significant differences by age were found for the other anxiety disorders. The odds for boys to have a primary diagnosis of anxiety disorder was 2.63 (95% CI 1.52, 4.55), with a risk of 1.87 in children (95% CI 1.29, 2.72) and 0.71 in adolescents (95% CI 0.59, 0.86).

Among the participants that met the diagnosis criteria for at least one comorbidity (N = 194), adolescents were more likely than children to meet criteria for other anxiety disorder (14.7 vs. 13.6%, chi-square = 5.41; p = 0.02) or MDD (25.6 vs. 10.2%, chi-square = 5.49; p = 0.019). When looking at the age and gender trends for these comorbidities, we can observe some differences. While for the comorbidity with other anxiety disorder, the prevalence in adolescent boys is decreasing; in

		Children			Adolescents			Statistic
		Male (N = 60)	Female (N = 28)	All (N = 88)	Male (N = 70)	Female (N = 86)	All (N = 156)	(Children vs. adolescents)
Anxiety disorders	F40.0—(AG)	1 (1.7%)	1 (3.6%)	2	2 (2.9%)	0	2	$\chi^2(1) = 1.33, p = .24$
	F40.1—(SOC)	7 (11.7%)	3 (10.7%)	10	13 (18.6%)	7 (8.1%)	20	$\chi^2(1) = 0.75, p = .78$
	F40.2—(SPEC)	5 (8.3%)	5 (17.9%)	10	5 (7.1%)	0	5	$\chi^2(1) = 3.75, p = .05$
	F40.8—(NOS)	3 (5%)	4 (14.3%)	7	2 (2.9%)	3 (3.5%)	5	$\chi^2(1) = 0.01, p = .92$
	F40.9—(UNS)	0	1 (3.6%)	1	0	1 (1.2%)	1	—
	F41.0—(PD)	1 (1.7%)	0	1	3 (4.3%)	4 (4.7%)	7	$\chi^2(1) = 1.14, p = .28$
	F41.1—(GAD)	20 (33.3%)	5 (17.9%)	25	23 (32.9%)	39 (45.3%)	62	$\chi^2(1) = 13.11, p = .000$
	F41.2—(MAD)	7 (11.7%)	0	7	7 (10%)	14 (16.3%)	21	$\chi^2(1) = 9.33, p = .002$
	F41.3—(OMAD)	0	1 (3.6%)	1	0	3 (3.5%)	3	—
	F41.8—(OSA)	3 (5%)	0	3	8 (11.4%)	11 (12.8%)	19	$\chi^2(1) = 3.47, p = .06$
	F41.9—(ADU)	2 (3.3%)	0	2	5 (7.1%)	2 (2.3%)	7	$\chi^2(1) = 0.73, p = .39$
	F93.0—(SAD)	11 (18.3%)	8	19	1 (1.4%)	1 (1.7%)	2	$\chi^2(1) = 0.046, p = .83$
	F93.2—(SADC)	0	0	0	1 (1.4%)	1 (1.7%)	2	—
Comorbid anxiety disorders		8 (13.3%)	4 (14.3%)	12	6 (8.6%)	17 (19.8%)	23	$\chi^2(1) = 5.41, p = .02$

		Children			Adolescents			Statistic
		Male ($N = 60$)	**Female ($N = 28$)**	**All ($N = 88$)**	**Male ($N = 70$)**	**Female ($N = 86$)**	**All ($N = 156$)**	**(Children vs. adolescents)**
Mood disorder	MDD	7 (11.7%)	2 (7.1%)	9	14 (20%)	26 (30.2%)	40	$\chi^2(1) = 5.49, p = .019$
Other	ADHD	31 (51.7%)	13 (46.4%)	44	18 (25.7%)	8 (9.3%)	26	$\chi^2(1) = 0.012, p = .91$
	ASD	6 (10%)	4 (14.3%)	10	10 (14.3%)	1 (1.2%)	11	$\chi^2(1) = 2.75, p = .097$
	MR	3 (5%)	1 (3.6%)	4	4 (5.7%)	1 (1.2%)	5	—
	OCD	0	1 (3.6%)	1	1 (1.4%)	2 (2.3%)	3	—
	Conduct disorder	0	0	0	1 (1.4%)	1 (1.2%)	2	—
	ODD	1 (1.7%)	0	1	0	1 (1.2%)	1	—
	ATP	0	0	0	0	1 (1.2%)	1	
No disorder		4 (6.7%)	3 (10.7%)	7	15 (21.4%)	28 (32.6%)	43	$\chi^2(1) = 1.26, p = .261$

Note: AG = agoraphobia; SOC = social phobias; SPEC = specific phobias; NOS = other phobic anxiety disorders; UNS = phobic anxiety disorder, unspecified; PD = panic disorder; GAD = generalized anxiety disorder; MAD = mixed anxiety and depressive disorder; OMAD = other mixed anxiety disorders; OSA = other specified anxiety disorders; ADU = anxiety disorder, unspecified; SAD = separation anxiety disorder of childhood; SADC = social anxiety disorder of childhood; OAD = other anxiety disorders; MDD = major depressive disorder; ADHD = attention deficit hyperactivity disorder; CD = conduct disorder; ASD = autism spectrum disorder; MR = mental retardation; OCD = obsessive-compulsive disorder; ODD = oppositional defiant disorder; ATP = acute and transient psychotic disorders.

Table 1.
Child/adolescent primary anxiety disorder and comorbidities.

Anxiety disorders	OAD (*N* = 35)	MDD (*N* = 49)	ADHD (*N* = 70)	ASD (*N* = 21)	MD (*N* = 10)	ODD/CD (*N* = 5)	No disorder (*N* = 50)
F40.0—(AG)	1 (25%)	0	2 (50%)	0	0	0	1 (25%)
F40.1—(SOC)	4 (13.3%)	9 (30%)	10 (33.3%)	1 (3.3%)	1 (3.3%)	1 (3.3%)	4 (13.3%)
F40.2—(SPEC)	1 (6.7%)	1 (6.7%)	7 (46.7%)	3 (20%)	2 (13.3%)	0	1 (6.7%)
F40.8—(NOS)	2 (16.7%)	0	7 (58.3%)	0	0	0	2 (16.7%)
F40.9—(UNS)	0	0	1 (50%)	1 (50%)	0	0	0
F41.0—(PD)	1 (12.5%)	3 (37.5%)	0	0	1 (12.5%)	0	3 (37.5%)
F41.1—(GAD)	21 (24.1%)	22 (25.3%)	18 (20.7%)	9 (10.3%)	0	2 (2.2%)	14 (16.1%)
F41.2—(MAD)	3 (10.7%)	2 (7.1%)	8 (28.6%)	1 (3.6%)	0	1 (3.6%)	13 (45.4%)
F41.3—(OMAD)	1 (25%)	1 (25%)	1 (25%)	0	0	0	1 (25%)
F41.8—(OSA)	0	7 (31.8%)	3 (13.6%)	1 (4.5%)	3 (13.6%)	0	7 (31.8%)
F41.9—(ADU)	0	4 (44.4%)	1 (11.1%)	3 (33.3%)	0	0	1 (11.1%)
F93.0—(SAD)	1 (4.8%)	0	12 (57.1%)	2 (9.5%)	3 (14.3%)	1 (4.8%)	1 (4.8%)
F93.2—(SADC)	0	0	0	0	0	0	2 (100%)

Note: AG = agoraphobia; SOC = social phobias; SPEC = specific phobias; NOS = other phobic anxiety disorders; UNS = phobic anxiety disorder, unspecified; PD = panic disorder; GAD = generalized anxiety disorder; MAD = mixed anxiety and depressive disorder; OMAD = other mixed anxiety disorders; OSA = other specified anxiety disorders; ADU = anxiety disorder, unspecified; SAD = separation anxiety disorder of childhood; SADC = social anxiety disorder of childhood; OAD = other anxiety disorders; MDD = major depressive disorder; ADHD = attention deficit hyperactivity disorder; CD = conduct disorder; ASD = autism spectrum disorder; MR = mental retardation; ODD = oppositional defiant disorder.

Table 2.
Comorbidity patterns by principal diagnosis [percentage].

Anxiety disorders	Fluoxetine ($N = 23$)	Sertraline ($N = 65$)	Risperidone ($N = 25$)	Benzodiazepine ($N = 38$)	Other antipsychotics ($N = 22$)	Mood stabilizers ($N = 18$)	No pharmacological treatment ($N = 116$)
F40.0—(AG)	2 (50%)	1 (25%)	0	1 (25%)	0	0	1 (25%)
F40.1—(SOC)	2 (6.7%)	5 (16.7)	2 (6.7%)	2 (6.7%)	1 (3.3%)	0	21 (70%)
F40.2—(SPEC)	0	1 (6.7%)	3 (20%)	2 (13.3%)	1 (6.7%)	1 (6.7%)	10 (66.7%)
F40.8—(NOS)	0	4 (33.3%)	2 (16.7%)	1 (8.3%)	2 (16.6%)	5 (41.7%)	4 (33.3%)
F40.9—(UNS)	0	1 (50%)	0	0	0	0	1 (50%)
F41.0—(PD)	3 (37.5%)	4 (50%)	1 (12.5%)	4 (50%)	1 (12.5%)	0	0
F41.1—(GAD)	12 (13.8%)	30 (34.5%)	7 (8%)	19 (21.8%)	13 (14.9%)	6 (6.9%)	32 (36.8%)
F41.2—(MAD)	2 (7.1%)	7 (25%)	3 (10.7%)	1 (3.6%)	1 (3.6%)	4 (14.2%)	13 (46.4%)
F41.3—(OMAD)	0	0	0	1 (25%)	0	0	3 (75%)
F41.8—(OSA)	0	8 (36.4%)	3 (13.6%)	5 (22.7%)	2 (9%)	0	10 (45.5%)
F41.9—(ADU)	1 (11.1)	2 (22.2%)	2 (22.2%)	0	1 (11.1%)	0	4 (44.4%)
F93.0—(SAD)	1 (4.8%)	1 (4.8%)	2 (9.5%)	1 (4.8%)	0	0	17 (81%)
F93.2—(SADC)	0	1 (50%)	0	1 (50%)	0	2 (100%)	0

Note: AG = agoraphobia; SOC = social phobias; SPEC = specific phobias; NOS = other phobic anxiety disorders; UNS = phobic anxiety disorder, unspecified; PD = panic disorder; GAD = generalized anxiety disorder; MAD = mixed anxiety and depressive disorder; OMAD = other mixed anxiety disorders; OSA = other specified anxiety disorders; ADU = anxiety disorder, unspecified; SAD = separation anxiety disorder of childhood; SADC = social anxiety disorder of childhood.

Table 3.
Pharmacological treatment patterns by principal diagnosis (percentage).

adolescent girls it rises, being accountable for the significant difference between children and adolescents. For the comorbidity with MDD, the prevalence trends regarding age and sex are different than those for anxiety disorders. The comorbidity with MDD is rising with age, disregarding the gender, mentioning that the prevalence of MDD is higher in boys and the increase with age is milder than in girls.

There were no statistically significant relationships between the primary anxiety disorder diagnosis and gender. Regarding the comorbid diagnosis, the girls were more likely to receive an additional diagnosis of other anxiety disorder (18.4 vs. 10.8%), MDD (24.6 vs. 16.2%), while the boys were more likely to receive an additional diagnosis of ADHD (37.7 vs. 18.4%), ASD (12.3 vs. 4.4%), or MR (6.2 vs. 1.8%).

A chi-square analysis demonstrated that there was a significant difference in the presence of comorbidities between the principal diagnosis categories (chi-square = 132.46; p = .08). The principal anxiety disorders diagnosis with a higher number of comorbidities were GAD, SOC, MAD, OSA, and SAD, as seen in **Table 2**. Comorbidities associated with anxiety disorders are very common, especially among them. Patients with anxiety disorders had also high rates of depression and ADHD.

About 92% of the children and 72.4% of the adolescents with a primary diagnosis of anxiety disorder had at least one comorbidity, underlining that in our sample, the children had more comorbidities than the adolescents. The pattern of comorbidities was different for the most frequent anxiety disorders in our sample. For GAD, the most common comorbidities were other anxiety disorders and MDD, counting for almost half of the patients. Another 20.7% of them had comorbid ADHD. For MAD, the most frequent association was with ADHD, 28.6%, but the diagnosis includes specific symptoms of anxiety and depression, with neither type of symptom severe enough to justify a diagnosis if considered separately, so symptoms of depression are necessary for diagnosis. For SOC, the most frequent comorbidities were ADHD and MDD (~30%), followed by other anxiety disorders. SAD, which is a diagnosis specific for children, had comorbid ADHD in 57.1% of the cases.

From the 70 patients with ADHD comorbid diagnosis, 20 (28.6%) were treated with atomoxetine and 10 (14.3%) with methylphenidate. One hundred twenty-one (49.6%) patients in our sample didn't receive pharmacological treatment, 49 (55.7%) children and 72 (46.2%) adolescents, 65 (50%) boys and 56 (49.1%) girls (see **Table 3**). Seventy-five (30.7%) patients received only one medication, of which 30 (34.1%) children and 45 (28.8%) adolescents, 41 (31.5%) boys and 34 (29.8%) girls. Forty-eight patients received more than one pharmacological treatment, of which 9 (10.2%) were children and 39 (25%) were adolescents, 24 (18.5%) boys and 24 (21.1%) girls. There were no statistically significant relationships between the recommended treatment and gender, but there were significant differences regarding the age group (children vs. adolescents). A chi-square analysis demonstrated that there was a significant difference in mono and without versus more pharmacological treatments between children and adolescent categories (chi-square = 7.77; p = .02), the adolescents being more likely to receive more medication.

3. Discussion and conclusions

Anxiety disorders are considered to be the most common psychiatric disorder in children and adolescents. In our study out of 2471 patients assessed and/or treated in the Clinic of Pediatric Psychiatry from Cluj-Napoca, Romania, between January and December 2017, only 244 (9.88%) patients received a primary diagnosis of different anxiety disorders, meaning that the anxiety disorders were the reason for admission. This low frequency of anxiety disorders in a clinical sample of children and adolescents can be explained by the selection criteria but also by the fact that children internalization problems are less recognized by parents and referred for treatment. Merikangas et al. reported an overall prevalence of anxiety disorders with severe impairment and/or distress of 8.3%, which is close to the prevalence reported in our study [13]. In a meta-analysis of multiple data sets, Costello and Egger have found the prevalence of 10.2% for any AD, 5.4% for specific phobia (SPEC), 3.6% for social phobia (SOC), 2.6% for separation anxiety disorder (SAD), 1.7% for generalized anxiety disorder (GAD), and 0.8% for panic disorder (PD) [15]. In our sample, the prevalences for these disorders were 35.6% for GAD, 12.3% for SOC, 8.6% for SAD, 6.1% for SPEC, and 3.3% for PD.

The study results showed that 79.5% of the selected sample had a comorbid disorder, and 34.4% had an anxiety or mood comorbidity which is similar to the findings from other studies on comorbidity rates of anxiety disorders in children. Previous studies found constantly elevated comorbidity rates in people with anxiety disorders [43], associated with increased symptom severity and greater functional impairment and worse outcome [15, 44]. The Child/Adolescent Anxiety Multimodal Study (CAMS) identified children and adolescents with social phobia, GAD, or SAD. They found that 78.6% of the sample had two or more of those disorders, and 35.9% met criteria for all three diagnoses simultaneously [36]. Kendall et al. find a comorbidity rate of 55.3% in a sample of youth with anxiety disorders [45]. Costello et al. found that comorbidity of AD with other psychiatric disorders was common, varying from 53% for GAD to 100% for SPEC. The most common type of comorbidity with non-anxiety disorders was with depression [15]. Also, the association between GAD and depression was found by Moffitt et al. in the Dunedin, New Zealand, longitudinal study with GAD predicting depression and depression predicting GAD across the life course [46]. In our study, 83.9% of the patients diagnosed with GAD had comorbidities, and 50% of them were diagnosed also with other anxiety disorder or depression.

Comorbidity patterns varied by *ICD-10* diagnosis. The principal diagnoses associated with significantly elevated risk for a comorbid diagnosis were GAD, MAD, SOC, OSA, and SAD. The association between GAD and other anxiety/depressive disorders raised many questions regarding the need for more accurate description in order to increase the reliability and validity of this disorder [47]. For SOC, the highest rate of comorbidities was with depression and ADHD. OSA had the highest comorbidity rate with depression, MAD with other anxiety disorders and ADHD and SAD with ADHD.

In our study, the prevalence of anxiety disorders primary diagnosis was 9.88%, with slightly different rates in females (46.7%) and males (53.3%). Although there were a greater number of boys than girls included in the study, the situation was different on age groups, more boys than girls in children group and more girls than boys in adolescent group; gender was not significantly associated with any of the anxiety diagnosis or comorbidity. The most common disorders in both males and females were GAD, SOC, MAD, other specified anxiety disorders (OSA), and separation anxiety disorder of childhood (SAD). Adolescents were more likely to receive a principal diagnosis of GAD or MAD than children. The prevalences of generalized anxiety disorder (GAD) and mixed anxiety and depressive (MAD) disorder were found higher in adolescents than in children (see **Table 1**), but with a higher prevalence in adolescent girls, the proportion of boys diagnosed with GAD and MAD being relatively stable with age. Children were more likely to receive a principal diagnosis of SPEC than adolescents. For specific phobias (SPEC), the prevalence was higher in children than in adolescents, but while the proportion of boys remained relatively stable, the diagnosis wasn't present in adolescent girls. No significant differences by age were found for the other anxiety disorders.

Different anxiety disorders have different age and gender distributions during childhood and adolescence. Separation anxiety disorder (SAD) and specific phobias (SPEC) are more common in children, while panic disorder and social phobia are more common in adolescents. Recent studies showed that, in the general population, anxiety symptoms first decrease during early adolescence and subsequently increase from middle to late adolescence [22]. SAD and SPEC tend to emerge and predominate during childhood, whereas the initial onset of generalized anxiety disorder (GAD), panic disorder (PD), and social anxiety disorder (SAD) most often occurs during adolescence [24, 46].

According to the findings of our study, gender and age contributed to the presence of comorbidity. Adolescents were more likely than children to meet criteria for other anxiety disorder or MDD. The age and gender trends for these comorbidities were different. While for the comorbidity with other anxiety disorder, the prevalence in adolescent boys is decreasing; in adolescent girls, it rises, being accountable for the significant difference between children and adolescents. For the comorbidity with MDD, the prevalence trends regarding age and sex are different. The comorbidity with MDD is rising with age, disregarding the gender, mentioning that the prevalence of MDD is higher in boys and the increase with age is milder than in girls. The girls were more likely to receive an additional diagnosis of other anxiety disorder and MDD, while the boys were more likely to receive an additional diagnosis of ADHD, ASD, or MR. This pattern is consistent with other studies which have found either no difference between the sexes or greater rates of comorbidity in males [48]. When examined separately, no difference was found in the presence of comorbidity by sex, for the principal diagnoses, but there were significant differences by age. The fact that adolescents experience higher levels of comorbid depressive disorders is consistent with findings from a clinical population [49].

Regarding the treatment patterns, in our study, the most frequently recommended pharmacological treatment was SSRIs, 36% of the patients receiving fluoxetine or sertraline. Other recommended treatments were benzodiazepines recommended to 15.6% of the patients, antipsychotics recommended to 19.3%, and mood stabilizers recommended to 7.4% of them. About 49.6% of the patients in our sample did not receive pharmacological treatment, 30.7% patients received only one medication, and 19.7% received more than one pharmacological treatment. There were no statistically significant relationships between the recommended treatment and gender, but there were significant differences regarding the age group (children vs. adolescents), the adolescents being more likely to receive more medication. These results should be interpreted keeping in mind that the sample had a high rate of comorbidities (79.5%) and that the pharmacological treatment may target those disorders. There is some evidence that medication can be effective in treating anxiety in children and adolescents, at least on the short term. A recent meta-analysis showed anxiolytic medication to be associated with a significantly greater clinical response than placebo (58.1 vs. 31.5%). Selective serotonin reuptake inhibitors (SSRIs) are regarded as the pharmacological treatment of choice for anxiety disorders in children and adolescents because of their effectiveness and safety profile. It is important to note that benzodiazepines have not been systematically assessed in children and adolescents, and, in view of concerns about dependency and side effects, their use is not recommended. It is unclear if there is an age below which medication would be contraindicated and what the duration of treatment should be [36]. Understanding the common patterns of anxiety disorders comorbidities and its treatments has important implications for child anxiety disorders treatment planning. Whether comorbid conditions might increase the need for treatment or cause patients to respond more poorly to psychological or psychiatric interventions is an important research area. Future treatments might need to be adapted to better meet the needs of patients with commonly occurring comorbid conditions. This will help facilitate a better choice of existing treatments and may improve treatment outcomes.

It is important to consider the methodological limitations of the study which may impact the conclusions drawn based on this data. The age was considered within two categories, based on childhood and adolescence that can be seen as distinct developmental periods, and future studies should look at narrower age bands. Additionally, the sample included only admitted patients and excluded those receiving services in outpatient settings.

Conflict of interest

The authors declare that they have no conflict of interest.

Author details

Elena Predescu[1,2]*, Anna Boglarka Asztalos[2] and Roxana Șipoș[1,2]

1 Department of Neuroscience, Discipline of Psychiatry and Pediatric Psychiatry, "Iuliu Hatieganu" University of Medicine and Pharmacy, Cluj-Napoca, Romania

2 Clinical Emergency Hospital for Children Cluj-Napoca, Clinic of Pediatric Psychiatry, Cluj-Napoca, Romania

*Address all correspondence to: predescu.elena@umfcluj.ro

References

[1] American Psychiatric Association. Diagnostic and Statistical Manual of Mental Disorders. 5th ed. Washington, DC: American Psychiatric Association; 2013

[2] World Health Organization. The ICD-10 Classification of Mental and Behavioural Disorders: Clinical Descriptions and Diagnostic Guidelines. Geneva: World Health Organization; 1992

[3] Schniering CA, Hudson JL, Rapee RM. Issues in the diagnosis and assessment of anxiety disorders in children and adolescents. Clinical Psychology Review. 2000;**20**(4): 453-478. PMID: 10832549

[4] Rutter M, Uher R. Classification issues and challenges in child and adolescent psychopathology. International Review of Psychiatry. 2012;**24**:514-529

[5] Kogan CS, Stein DJ, Maj M, First MB, Emmelkamp PM, Reed GM. The classification of anxiety and fear-related disorders in the ICD-11. Depression and Anxiety. 2016;**33**(12):1141-1154. DOI: 10.1002/da.22530

[6] Muris P, Simon E, Lijphart H, Bos A, Hale W 3rd, Schmeitz K, et al. The youth anxiety measure for DSM-5 (YAM-5): Development and first psychometric evidence of a new scale for assessing anxiety disorders symptoms of children and adolescents. Child Psychiatry and Human Development. 2017;**48**(1):1-17. DOI: 10.1007/s10578-016-0648-1

[7] Möller EL, Majdandžić M, Craske MG, Bögels SM. Dimensional assessment of anxiety disorders in parents and children for DSM-5. International Journal of Methods in Psychiatric Research. 2014;**23**(3): 331-344. DOI: 10.1002/mpr.1450

[8] Rappaport BI, Pagliaccio D, Pine DS, Klein DN, Jarcho JM. Discriminant validity, diagnostic utility, and parent-child agreement on the screen for child anxiety related emotional disorders (SCARED) in treatment- and non-treatment-seeking youth. Journal of Anxiety Disorders. 2017;**51**:22-31. DOI: 10.1016/j.janxdis.2017.08.006

[9] Păsărelu CR, Dobrean A, Balazsi R, Predescu E, Şipos R, Lupu V. The Penn State worry questionnaire for children: Age, gender and clinical invariance. Child Psychiatry and Human Development. 2017;**48**(3):359-369. DOI: 10.1007/s10578-016-0663-2

[10] Lebeau RT, Glenn DE, Hanover LN, Beesdo-Baum K, Wittchen HU, Craske MG. A dimensional approach to measuring anxiety for DSM-5. International Journal of Methods in Psychiatric Research. 2012;**21**(4): 258-272. DOI: 10.1002/mpr.1369

[11] Schniering CA, Hudson JL, Rapee RM. Issues in the diagnosis and assessment of anxiety disorders in children and adolescents. Clinical Psychology Review. 2000;**20**(4): 453-478. PMID: 10832549

[12] Polanczyk GV, Salum GA, Sugaya LS, Caye A, Rohde LA. Annual research review: A meta-analysis of the worldwide prevalence of mental disorders in children and adolescents. Journal of Child Psychology and Psychiatry. 2015;**56**(3):345-365. DOI: 10.1111/jcpp.12381

[13] Merikangas KR, He JP, Burstein M, Swanson SA, Avenevoli S, Cui L, et al. Lifetime prevalence of mental disorders in U.S. adolescents: Results from the National Comorbidity Survey Replication—Adolescent Supplement (NCS-A). Journal of the American Academy of Child and Adolescent Psychiatry.

2010;**49**(10):980-989. DOI: 10.1016/j.jaac.2010.05.017

[14] Costello EJ, Egger H, Angold A. 10-year research update review: The epidemiology of child and adolescent psychiatric disorders: I. Methods and public health burden. Journal of the American Academy of Child and Adolescent Psychiatry. 2005;**44**(10):972-986. PMID: 16175102

[15] Costello E, Egger H, Copeland W, Erkanli A, Angold A. The developmental epidemiology of anxiety disorders: Phenomenology, prevalence, and comorbidity. In: Silverman W, Field A, editors. Anxiety Disorders in Children and Adolescents. Cambridge Child and Adolescent Psychiatry. Cambridge: Cambridge University Press; 2011. pp. 56-75. DOI: 10.1017/CBO9780511994920.004

[16] Kessler RC, Avenevoli S, Costello EJ, Georgiades K, Green JG, Gruber MJ, et al. Prevalence, persistence, and sociodemographic correlates of DSM-IV disorders in the National comorbidity survey replication adolescent supplement. Archives of General Psychiatry. 2012;**69**(4):372-380. DOI: 10.1001/archgenpsychiatry.2011.160

[17] Spence SH, Zubrick SR, Lawrence D. A profile of social, separation and generalized anxiety disorders in an Australian nationally representative sample of children and adolescents: Prevalence, comorbidity and correlates. The Australian and New Zealand Journal of Psychiatry. 2018;**52**(5):446-460. DOI: 10.1177/0004867417741981

[18] Abbo C, Kinyanda E, Kizza RB, Levin J, Ndyanabangi S, Stein DJ. Prevalence, comorbidity and predictors of anxiety disorders in children and adolescents in rural North-Eastern Uganda. Child and Adolescent Psychiatry and Mental Health. 2013;7(1):21. DOI: 10.1186/1753-2000-7-21

[19] Shea CKS, Lee MMC, Lai KYC, Luk ESL, Leung PWL. Prevalence of anxiety disorders in Hong Kong Chinese children with ADHD. Journal of Attention Disorders. 2018;**22**(5):403-413. DOI: 10.1177/1087054714562830

[20] Essau CA, Conradt J, Petermann F. Frequency, comorbidity, and psychosocial impairment of anxiety disorders in German adolescents. Journal of Anxiety Disorders. 2000;**14**(3):263-279. PMID: 10868984

[21] Kessler RC, Berglund P, Demler O, Jin R, Merikangas KR, Walters EE. Lifetime prevalence and age-of-onset distributions of DSM-IV disorders in the National comorbidity survey replication. Archives of General Psychiatry. 2005;**62**(6):593-602. Erratum in: Archives of General Psychiatry. 2005;62(7):768. Merikangas, Kathleen R [added]. PubMed PMID: 15939837

[22] Van Oort FV, Greaves-Lord K, Verhulst FC, Ormel J, Huizink AC. The developmental course of anxiety symptoms during adolescence: The TRAILS study. Journal of Child Psychology and Psychiatry. 2009;**50**(10):1209-1217. DOI: 10.1111/j.1469-7610.2009.02092.x

[23] Beesdo-Baum K, Knappe S. Developmental epidemiology of anxiety disorders. Child and Adolescent Psychiatric Clinics of North America. 2012;**21**(3):457-478. DOI: 10.1016/j.chc.2012.05.001

[24] Ohannessian CM, Milan S, Vannucci A. Gender differences in anxiety trajectories from middle to late adolescence. Journal of Youth and Adolescence. 2017;**46**(4):826-839. DOI: 10.1007/s10964-016-0619-7

[25] Crocetti E, Klimstra T, Keijsers L, Hale WW 3rd, Meeus W. Anxiety trajectories and identity development in adolescence: A five-wave longitudinal study. Journal of Youth and Adolescence. 2009;**38**(6):839-849. DOI: 10.1007/s10964-008-9302-y

[26] Nelemans SA, Hale WW, Branje SJ, Raaijmakers QA, Frijns T, van Lier PA, et al. Heterogeneity in development of adolescent anxiety disorder symptoms in an 8-year longitudinal community study. Development and Psychopathology. 2014;**26**(1):181-202. DOI: 10.1017/S0954579413000503

[27] Legerstee JS, Verhulst FC, Robbers SC, Ormel J, Oldehinkel AJ, van Oort FV. Gender-specific developmental trajectories of anxiety during adolescence: Determinants and outcomes. The TRAILS study. Journal of Canadian Academy of Child and Adolescent Psychiatry. 2013;**22**(1): 26-34. PMID: 23390430

[28] Merikangas KR, Nakamura EF, Kessler RC. Epidemiology of mental disorders in children and adolescents. Dialogues in Clinical Neuroscience. 2009;**11**(1):7-20. PMID: 19432384

[29] Hale WW 3rd, Raaijmakers Q, Muris P, van Hoof A, Meeus W. Developmental trajectories of adolescent anxiety disorder symptoms: A 5-year prospective community study. Journal of the American Academy of Child and Adolescent Psychiatry. 2008;**47**(5):556-564. DOI: 10.1097/CHI.0b013e3181676583

[30] McLaughlin KA, King K. Developmental trajectories of anxiety and depression in early adolescence. Journal of Abnormal Child Psychology. 2015;**43**(2):311-323. DOI: 10.1007/s10802-014-9898-1

[31] Stapinski LA, Araya R, Heron J, Montgomery AA, Stallard P. Peer victimization during adolescence: Concurrent and prospective impact on symptoms of depression and anxiety. Anxiety, Stress, and Coping. 2015;**28**(1):105-120. DOI: 10.1080/10615806.2014.962023

[32] Rapee RM, Schniering CA, Hudson JL. Anxiety disorders during childhood and adolescence: Origins and treatment. Annual Review of Clinical Psychology. 2009;**5**:311-341. DOI: 10.1146/annurev.clinpsy.032408.153628

[33] Waite P, Creswell C. Children and adolescents referred for treatment of anxiety disorders: Differences in clinical characteristics. Journal of Affective Disorders. 2014;**167**:326-332. DOI: 10.1016/j.jad.2014.06.028

[34] Rockhill C, Kodish I, DiBattisto C, Macias M, Varley C, Ryan S. Anxiety disorders in children and adolescents. Current Problems in Pediatric and Adolescent Health Care. 2010;**40**(4):66-99. DOI: 10.1016/j.cppeds.2010.02.002

[35] Schatz DB, Rostain AL. ADHD with comorbid anxiety: A review of the current literature. Journal of Attention Disorders. 2006;**10**(2):141-149. PMID: 17085624

[36] Walkup JT, Albano AM, Piacentini J, Birmaher B, Compton SN, Sherrill JT, et al. Cognitive behavioral therapy, sertraline, or a combination in childhood anxiety. The New England Journal of Medicine. 2008;**359**(26): 2753-2766. DOI: 10.1056/NEJMoa0804633

[37] Hankin BL, Snyder HR, Gulley LD, Schweizer TH, Bijttebier P, Nelis S, et al. Understanding comorbidity among internalizing problems: Integrating latent structural models of psychopathology and risk mechanisms. Development and Psychopathology. 2016;**28**(4pt1):987-1012. PMID: 27739389

[38] Copeland WE, Angold A, Shanahan L, Costello EJ. Longitudinal patterns of anxiety from childhood to adulthood: The Great Smoky Mountains study. Journal of the American Academy of Child and Adolescent Psychiatry. 2014;**53**(1):21-33. DOI: 10.1016/j.jaac.2013.09.017

[39] Lewinsohn P, Zinbarg J, Lewinsohn M, Sack W. Lifetime comorbidity among anxiety disorders and between anxiety disorders and other mental disorders in adolescents. Journal of Anxiety Disorders. 1997;**11**:377-394

[40] Sterba S, Egger HL, Angold A. Diagnostic specificity and nonspecificity in the dimensions of preschool psychopathology. Journal of Child Psychology and Psychiatry. 2007;**48**(10):1005-1013. PMID: 17915001

[41] Essau CA, Conradt J, Petermann F. Frequency and comorbidity of social phobia and social fears in adolescents. Behaviour Research and Therapy. 1999;**37**(9):831-843. DOI: 10.1016/S0005-7967(98)00179-X

[42] Ramsawh HJ, Raffa SD, Edelen MO, Rende R, Keller MB. Anxiety in middle adulthood: Effects of age and time on the 14-year course of panic disorder, social phobia and generalized anxiety disorder. Psychological Medicine. 2009;**39**(4):615-624. DOI: 10.1017/S0033291708003954

[43] Kendall PC, Compton SN, Walkup JT, Birmaher B, Albano AM, Sherrill J, et al. Clinical characteristics of anxiety disordered youth. Journal of Anxiety Disorders. 2010;**24**(3):360-365

[44] Moffitt TE, Harrington H, Caspi A, Kim-Cohen J, Goldberg D, Gregory AM, et al. Depression and generalized anxiety disorder: Cumulative and sequential comorbidity in a birth cohort followed prospectively to age 32 years. Archives of General Psychiatry. 2007;**64**:651-660

[45] Moffitt TE, Caspi A, Taylor A, Kokaua J, Milne BJ, Polanczyk G, et al. How common are common mental disorders? Evidence that lifetime prevalence rates are doubled by prospective versus retrospective ascertainment. Psychological Medicine. 2010;**40**(6):899-909. DOI: 10.1017/S0033291709991036

[46] Masi G, Millepiedi S, Mucci M, Poli P, Bertini N, Milantoni L. Generalized anxiety disorder in referred children and adolescents. Journal of the American Academy of Child and Adolescent Psychiatry. 2004;**43**(6):752-760. PubMed PMID: 15167092

[47] Strauss CC, Last CG, Hersen M, Kazdin AE. Association between anxiety and depression in children and adolescents with anxiety disorders. Journal of Abnormal Child Psychology. 1988;**16**(1):57-68. PMID: 3361030

[48] Ipser JC, Stein DJ, Hawkridge S, Hoppe L. Pharmacotherapy for anxiety disorders in children and adolescents. Cochrane Database of Systematic Reviews. 2009;**8**(3):CD005170. DOI: 10.1002/14651858.CD005170

[49] Brown AM, Deacon BJ, Abramowitz JS, Dammann J, Whiteside SP. Parents' perceptions of pharmacological and for childhood anxiety disorders. Behaviour Research and Therapy. 2007;**45**(4):819-828. PMID: 16784722

Section 2

Anxiety as Modulator of Life

Chapter 7

A Meta-Analysis of Sleep Disturbances in Panic Disorder

Geneviève Belleville and Alenka Potočnik

Abstract

The nature and prevalence of sleep disturbances in panic disorder (PD) have been often discussed but remain unclear. The objective of this systematic review and meta-analysis is to document sleep disturbances in PD. Systematic database search and standardized extraction were conducted. Meta-analysis was computed on self-report (subjective) and polysomnographic (PSG) (objective) data and on prevalence rates of nocturnal panic attacks (NPA). Of the 1262 publications retrieved, 31 were included. PD patients were compared to healthy controls on subjective and objective measures. Patients had higher Pittsburgh sleep quality index (PSQI) global scores (hedges' g = 1.306, 95% CI [0.532, 2.081]), longer PSG sleep latency (hedges' g = 0.81, 95% CI [0.576, 1.035]), poorer PSG sleep efficiency (hedges' g = −0.79, 95% CI [−1.124, −0.432]), and shorter stage 2 (hedges' g = 0.70, 95% CI [−1.231, −0.120]) and total sleep time (hedges' g = −0.739, 95% CI [−1.127, −0.351]). Among patients, 52.1% (95% CI [0.464, 0.577]) reported NPA (≥1/lifetime). Patients with PD demonstrate subjective and objective sleep alterations. More than half have experienced NPA. These sleep disturbances could have a significant role in maintaining PD symptoms.

Keywords: panic disorder, nocturnal panic attacks, insomnia, sleep, sleep disturbances, meta-analysis

1. Introduction

Panic disorder (PD) is a common anxiety disorder, with a prevalence rate of 3.7% in the general population [1]. It is characterized by sudden and recurrent surges of anxiety known as panic attacks, apprehensiveness about panic, and avoidance of potential future panic attacks [2]. In PD, as in many anxiety disorders [3], sleep may be affected. The existing literature describes two primary types of sleep problems in patients with PD: insomnia and nocturnal panic attacks (NPA).

1.1 Insomnia in patients with PD

DSM-IV-TR defines insomnia as difficulty initiating or maintaining sleep, early awakening, or non-restorative sleep [4]. Symptoms must be present at least three times per week for at least 1 month and must be the source of significant distress or dysfunction [4]. Compared to DSM-IV-TR, DSM-5 added new criteria for insomnia, including early awakening and dissatisfaction with sleep quality [2]. Furthermore, the minimum duration of symptoms was increased to 3 months [2]. Insomnia is assessed using a wide variety of measures that can be generally classified as subjective or objective. The former uses self-report questionnaires and diaries or clinician-rated assessments; the latter uses physiological measures such as polysomnography or actigraphy [5].

1.2 Nocturnal panic attacks

NPA are paroxysmal events characterized by abrupt awakening in a state of intense anxiety and discomfort [6]. In contrast with panic attacks that begin after waking, individuals experiencing NPA wake up in a state of panic [2]. Nocturnal panic attacks generally occur between stage 2 and stage 3 sleep and are not associated with the content of a nightmare [6]. In the majority of cases, daytime panic attacks are more frequent than NPA. However, a minority of patients primarily experience nocturnal panic attacks [7], and cases of individuals with exclusively nocturnal panic attacks have been reported [8]. Nocturnal panic attacks can be assessed using the NPA appendix from the anxiety disorders interview schedule for DSM-IV. This clinician-administered interview thoroughly assesses NPA and includes questions relating to NPA frequency, apprehensiveness about future NPA, and avoidance behaviors.

1.3 Why study sleep in panic disorder?

Disturbed sleep in patients with PD is associated with greater PD severity [9]. In a recent study, researchers found that there was a significantly higher prevalence of insomnia (insomnia severity index > 8) in patients with severe or moderate PD symptoms than in patients with mild symptoms [9]. In addition to being associated with symptom severity, sleep disturbances, specifically NPA, are associated with suicidal behavior [10].

Not only are sleep disturbances (insomnia and NPA) associated with greater PD severity and with suicidal behavior, they are also hypothesized to perpetuate panic symptoms. Researchers have proposed that insomnia, NPA, and panic interact and reinforce one another in a vicious cycle [11]. Studies of individuals from the general population revealed that one night of sleep deprivation increases general anxiety and physiological activation [12]. In a similar experiment with patients with PD, researchers observed panic attacks in 40% of patients after one night of sleep deprivation, although none of the participants had experienced a panic attack in the prior week [13]. In the same study, none of the control participants (healthy controls or patients with obsessive-compulsive disorder) reported a panic attack the following day [13]. Although the experience of insomnia is distinct from the experience of sleep deprivation, patients with chronic insomnia can develop a sleep deficit [14]. Some researchers have therefore hypothesized that the effect of chronic insomnia could be comparable (although less intense) to the effect of sleep deprivation, resulting in increased general activation and triggering panic attacks [11]. When an individual also experiences NPA, they may develop apprehensiveness about going to sleep [15]. Apprehensiveness can result in a delayed bedtime, thereby compounding lack of sleep, increasing general activation, and potentially triggering panic [11]. Furthermore, some patients with PD tend to experience distress and even panic attacks in states of relaxation or states of decreased vigilance [16, 17]. It is hypothesized that such a reaction may occur immediately prior to sleep in some patients and may disturb sleep onset.

1.4 Unresolved issues related to insomnia in patients with PD

1.4.1 Subjective sleep data

Numerous studies have reported subjective sleep data from patients with PD, collected using a wide variety of psychometric tools. For example, many studies have used the Pittsburgh sleep quality index and report a general sleep quality index [18–21]. The Hamilton depression scale (HAM-D) is another frequently used scale that assesses difficulty initiating and maintaining sleep, as well as early awakenings [22–25]. Moreover, some studies measure variables that are not included in the definition of insomnia, such as sleep duration [23]. This diversity of variables and measures complexifies comparison between studies and precludes a clear portrait of sleep alterations in PD.

1.4.2 Objective sleep data

In contrast to subjective sleep data, objective data is collected in a standardized fashion, generating results that are comparable across studies. However, despite greater uniformity in assessment, the literature on objective sleep data has yielded contradictory results. For example, some authors have reported poorer sleep efficiency in patients with PD in comparison to healthy controls [19, 26], whereas others report no difference between groups [27]. Similarly, inconsistent results have been published about slow-wave sleep (stages 3 and 4) and REM sleep latency [6, 22, 26–31]. The wealth of conflicting data is confusing and can lead to erroneous conclusions. For example, if two studies report a difference between PD and control groups in a given variable and two others report no difference, readers tend to conclude that no substantial difference exists, which may not be the case [32]. Among possible explanations, inconsistencies may be partly attributable to a lack of statistical power: indeed, polysomnographic studies tend to have small sample sizes due to their costly and complex nature.

1.5 Unresolved issues concerning the prevalence of NPA in patients with PD

The results of NPA prevalence studies vary significantly. For example, Schredl et al. [33] reported an NPA prevalence rate of 37%, whereas Stein et al. [20] reported a figure almost twice as high (68%). Moreover, different authors use different frequency criteria, ranging from "at least one lifetime NPA" [34–36], to "two to four NPA per year" [33], to "a minimum of four NPA per month" [37], or to "many times per week" [33]. A summary of the data is indicated in order to gain clarity on the rate of NPA in patients with PD.

1.6 The need for a systematic literature review and meta-analysis

The unanswered questions described above indicate a clear need for a more precise portrait of sleep disturbances in PD. A systematic review of the existing literature is warranted. Some authors have undertaken the effort in recent decades [38–41], but contradictory results from objective data and variations in the reporting of subjective data resulted in questions remaining about sleep alterations in the population. Lack of uniformity in NPA prevalence measurement and reporting yielded significant variability in prevalence rate estimates. Meta-analytic methodology involves pooling all samples into one group to conduct a quantitative analysis of data from previous research, with greater statistical power than when analyzing each study's data alone. This method would likely allow for a clearer interpretation of the current literature on the subject.

The present study was designed to systematically review the existing literature on sleep disturbances in PD. More precisely, the objectives were (1) to compare sleep in patients with PD to sleep in healthy controls and (2) to assess the prevalence rate of NPA in patients with PD. We hypothesized that the sleep of patients with PD would be significantly different from that of healthy controls.

2. Method

The preferred reporting items for systematic reviews and meta-analysis (PRISMA) checklist was used to design the study and to report results based on best practices in the field of literature reviews and meta-analyses [42].

2.1 Literature research

We conducted a literature review in these databases: PsycNet, MedLine, ProQuest, Web of Knowledge, Cochrane, and Psychology and Behavioral Sciences Collection. Search terms used in PsycNet were "panic disorder" OR "panic attack" OR panic AND sleep OR "sleep disorders" OR insomnia OR "nocturnal panic" OR "sleep deprivation." Search terms used in MedLine, Web of Knowledge, and Cochrane were panic OR "panic disorder" AND sleep OR "sleep initiation and maintenance disorders" OR dyssomnia OR "sleep deprivation." Publication date was 1980 (DSM-III year of publication) to May 2016 inclusive.

To retrieve gray literature (i.e., unpublished work or studies that are published outside widely available journals) [43], reference lists of selected articles were searched for potentially eligible articles regarding sleep in PD. The Laval University library was searched for book chapters addressing sleep in PD. Reference lists were screened for articles of interest. Inclusion of ProQuest and Web of Knowledge databases helped retrieve gray literature, as these sources contain theses, symposia, and convention papers, in addition to journal articles.

2.2 Article selection

The following inclusion criteria were used: (a) studies had to be published in English, French, or Spanish; (b) minimum participant age was 18 years; (c) to ensure population representativeness, studies including participants with comorbidities were accepted if PD was the primary diagnosis for at least one subgroup; (d) studies had to report quantitative group data for at least one sleep variable; (e) data on sleep disturbances had to include means, standard deviations, and group sizes for PD and control groups; (f) prevalence of NPA had to be reported in percentage or number of participants, and total sample size had to be included; (g) data had to be issued from self-report questionnaires, clinician-administered interviews, sleep diaries, polysomnography, or actigraphy; and (h) for subjective and objective sleep data, patients with PD had to be compared to a group of healthy controls (for the prevalence of nocturnal panic, no comparison group was necessary).

Studies that met the following criterion were excluded: (a) studies in which all patients with PD reported a physical disease or one of the following comorbid psychiatric disorders, schizophrenia, bipolar disorder, and alcohol or drug abuse or dependence, and (b) studies in which no data could be grouped using the following procedure:

Studies were classified and grouped on the basis of the measure they reported. For example, all studies reporting results on the Pittsburgh sleep quality index (PSQI) were grouped together, the same was done for the Hamilton rating scale (HAM-D), polysomnography, etc. For articles reporting NPA, grouping was carried out on the basis of the frequency criteria used. For example, all studies reporting the prevalence of patients who had at least one NPA in their lifetime were grouped together, all articles reporting the prevalence of patients having at least one NPA/month were grouped together, etc. Some articles reported data from specific sleep measures or NPA frequency criteria that were not repeated elsewhere.

Studies reporting data that could not be grouped with other data from at least one additional study were excluded.

2.3 Data extraction

Once reference retrieval was complete, each of the selected papers was reviewed, and data was extracted using a standardized rating form and coding manual. Extracted variables included information about the sample and sampling method, general methodology, and sleep characteristics (self-report sleep data, polysomnographic/actigraphic data, and prevalence of NPA).

2.4 Inter-rater agreement

2.4.1 Article selection

To reduce selection bias, a second trained judge independently rated the eligibility of 30% of the retrieved literature. The results of the two judges' ratings were compared, and cases of disagreement were discussed to reach consensus.

2.4.2 Data extraction

Five raters participated in data extraction. Four of the judges were undergraduate psychology students, and one was a graduate psychology student (AP). A pilot coding was conducted, wherein all judges used the coding manual to rate the same

Item	Percentage inter-rater agreement
Study description	
PD group sample size	100.0
Control group sample size	100.0
Mean age	88.2
Gender	73.1
Medication permitted or not	96.2
Percentage of participants taking medication	84.6
Psychometric instrument used to diagnose PD	82.7
Psychometric instrument used to assess sleep	100.0
Self-report data	
Sleep variable—PD group	88.9
Sleep variable—control group	88.9
Polysomnographic data	
Sleep variable—PD group	100.0
Sleep variable—control group	98.8
NPA	
Percentage of sample reporting NPA	46.7
NPA frequency criterion	66.7

Note: NPA = nocturnal panic attack; PD = panic disorder.

Table 1.
Inter-rater agreement.

four studies. When training was complete, studies were randomly assigned to one of the four undergraduate judges. The graduate student acted as second judge and independently coded all studies. Regular meetings were held to review discrepancies and reach consensus. In total, 29 of the 31 studies (93.5%) included in the meta-analysis were independently rated by two judges. The percentages of inter-rater agreement were between 70 and 100% for the majority of coded variables (see details in **Table 1**). Lower agreement rates were observed on variables related to NPA, a finding that can be explained by a lack of precision in reports of NPA prevalence.

2.5 Data analysis

Results were analyzed using the comprehensive meta-analysis software, version 3. Since the studies included in this review varied widely, a random effects model was used. Many of the studies had small sample sizes, in particular polysomnographic studies. Hedges' g was consequently chosen for effect size because of its correction for small samples [32]. Q and I^2 were used to assess heterogeneity. For each analysis of significant results including three studies or more, Orwin's fail-safe N was used to investigate publication bias. In these cases, a funnel plot was visually examined.

3. Results

A total of 1229 articles were screened for eligibility (**Figure 1**). Of the 1229,80 initially met inclusion criteria. Forty-nine were subsequently excluded. A total of 31 studies were selected for review. The majority of studies with self-report or polysomnographic data reported no significant differences in age or gender ratio

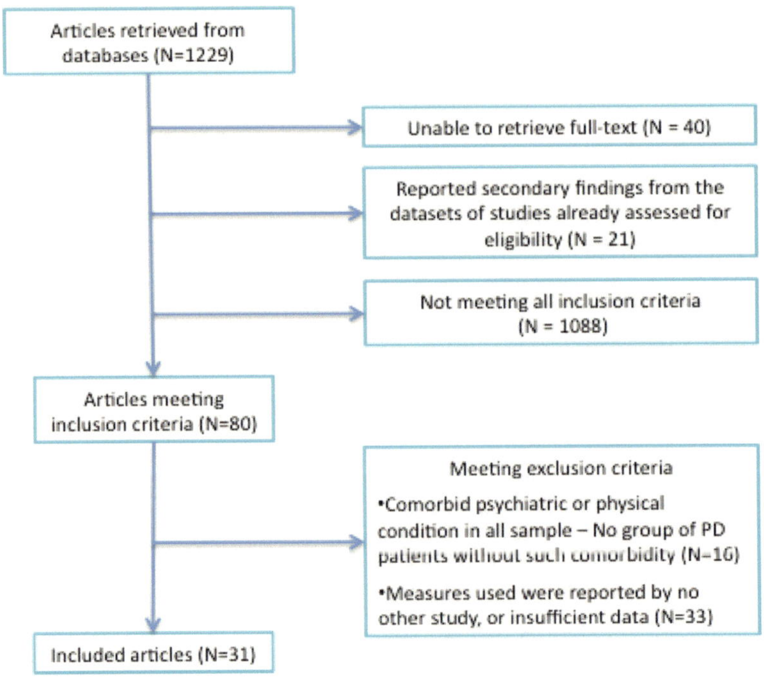

Figure 1.
Study selection flow chart.

between PD and control groups. Of the 31 studies analyzed, seven included participants taking medication. Participants were medication-free in all but one of the polysomnographic studies. In all studies, PD diagnoses were made using validated diagnostic interviews. The majority of patient samples were recruited in clinics/hospitals or were referred by a health professional. Control participants were mostly recruited through local media.

3.1 Self-report sleep data

Of the 31 selected articles, seven reported self-report data. All seven studies used the PSQI. The component scales of subjective sleep quality, sleep latency, sleep duration, sleep efficiency, sleep disturbances, daytime dysfunction, and the PSQI global score were analyzed. The sixth PSQI scale (medication use) was not analyzed because the variable was outside the scope of the present study. Pooled PD group size ranged from 47 to 182 participants (average = 94 participants). Pooled control groups ranged from 15,151 to 15,238 participants (average = 15,163 participants) (**Table 2**). The wide difference between average group size in PD and control groups was due to the presence of one study whose control group was 15,117 participants. When this study was removed from calculations of the average sample size, average control group size was 46 participants.

Analyses revealed that patients with PD had significantly greater scores than healthy controls for the PSQI scales of sleep quality, sleep latency, sleep disturbances, daily dysfunction, and global score. This means that patients with PD reported worse sleep quality, longer sleep latency, more sleep disturbances, and more daily dysfunction. All effect sizes were large as per Cohen's criteria [44]. There were no significant differences between groups on PSQI sleep efficiency and sleep duration scales.

Variable	Effect size (Hedges' g)	95% CI	Standard error	Variance	Q	I^2	Number of studies	PD group sample size	Control group sample size
PSQI subjective sleep quality	1.76*	[1.26, 2.31]	0.28	0.08	—	—	2	89	15,151
PSQI sleep latency	1.31*	[0.42, 2.21]	0.46	0.21	—	—	2	89	15,151
PSQI sleep duration	−0.18	[−1.33, 0.98]	0.59	0.35	—	—	2	89	15,151
PSQI sleep efficiency	0.81	[−0.08, 1.70]	0.45	0.21	—	—	2	89	15,151
PSQI sleep disturbances	1.56*	[0.65, 2.47]	0.46	0.22	—	—	2	89	15,151
PSQI daily dysfunction	1.71*	[1.38, 2.04]	0.17	0.03	—	—	2	89	15,151
PSQI global score	1.31*	[0.53, 2.08]	0.40	0.16	69.38**	92.79	6	182	15,238

Note: PSQI = Pittsburgh sleep quality index; — = insufficient number of studies to report heterogeneity; CI = confidence interval.
**= Significant differences between groups, $p < 0.05$.*
***= Significant heterogeneity, $p < 0.05$.*

Table 2.
Meta-analysis results for self-report data.

To evaluate the consistency of data across studies, heterogeneity tests were performed on data for PSQI global score. The results indicated the presence of significant heterogeneity. Estimated variance in true effects (I^2) was 92.8%. The small number of effect sizes precluded subgroup or meta-regression analyses that may have explained the heterogeneity of results.

Among subjective sleep variables, the impact of publication bias was assessed for PSQI global score. Results of Orwin's fail-safe N indicated that 48 unpublished studies with no effect would be required to lower the combined effect for PSQI global score to 0.2 (criterion for trivial effect). Moreover, the analysis of the funnel plot revealed an uneven distribution of studies, the majority of which were below the mean Hedges' g value. That is, both Orwin's fail-safe N and funnel plot analysis suggest the possibility of publication bias due to a "file drawer effect" (i.e., fewer studies with unsignificant results are published). The results must therefore be interpreted with caution.

3.2 Polysomnographic sleep data

Of the 31 included studies, 15 reported polysomnographic or actigraphic data. Meta-analysis was performed with 18 variables: sleep latency, sleep efficiency, number of awakenings, total sleep time, total wake time, REM sleep characteristics (duration, density, percentage, latency, number of REM periods), slow-wave sleep characteristics (duration, percentage), duration of stage 1 and stage 2 sleep, and percentage of stages 1–4 sleep. Pooled samples sizes varied between 19 and 209 participants for PD groups (average = 115 participants) and between 19 and 164 participants for control groups (average = 86 participants) (**Table 3**).

Significant differences between PD and control groups were demonstrated for four variables. PD participants had longer sleep latency, lower sleep efficiency, and shorter total sleep time than healthy controls. Duration of stage 2 sleep was also shorter. Analyses for the 14 other sleep variables did not show statistical significance.

To evaluate the consistency of data across studies, heterogeneity tests were performed on data for sleep latency, sleep efficiency, and total sleep time. The results indicated the presence of significant heterogeneity for sleep efficiency and for total sleep time. For the former, estimated variance in true effects (I^2) was 52%. For the latter, estimated variance in true effects (I^2) was 68%. There was no significant heterogeneity among sleep latency effect sizes. The small number of effect sizes precluded subgroup or meta-regression analyses that may have explained the heterogeneity of results.

We assessed the possibility of publication bias for the following variables: sleep latency, sleep efficiency, and total sleep time. For sleep latency, Orwin's fail-safe N was 31 (criterion for trivial Hedges' g = 0.2). This statistic indicates that it would take 31 studies with no effect to decrease the effect size to 0.2 or lower. Similar analysis yielded Orwin's fail-safe N of 26 for sleep efficiency and 24 for total sleep time. The results indicated that total effect size for each variable could be affected by publication bias. However, analysis of funnel plots, which are relatively well-balanced, indicated a lower probability of publication bias. When Orwin's fail-safe N and funnel plot analysis are combined, the possibility of publication bias cannot be excluded.

3.3 Prevalence of NPA

Thirteen studies were included in the analysis of the prevalence of NPA in patients with PD. Data was classified into three distinct categories according to

Variable	Effect size (Hedges'g)	Confidence interval (95%)	Standard error	Variance	Q	I^2	Number of studies	PD group sample size	Control group sample size
Sleep latency	0.81*	[0.58, 1.04]	0.12	0.01	7.95	0.00	10	168	147
Sleep efficiency	−0.78*	[−1.12, −0.43]	0.18	0.03	16.20**	50.62	9	186	118
Number of awakenings	0.07	[−0.25, 0.40]	0.17	0.03	2.35	0.00	4	80	66
Total sleep time	−0.74*	[−1.13, −0.35]	0.20	0.04	31.06**	67.80	11	209	164
Total wake time	0.58	[−0.20, 1.36]	0.40	0.16	27.02**	81.49	6	88	68
REM sleep duration	−0.12	[−0.75, 0.50]	0.32	0.10	4.15	51.76	4	65	51
REM sleep density	−0.04	[−0.41, 0.32]	0.19	0.03	1.73	0.00	4	64	52
% REM sleep	−0.01	[−0.22, 0.20]	0.11	0.01	6.98	0.00	10	181	134
REM latency	−0.25	[−0.73, 0.24]	0.25	0.06	33.48**	76.10	9	187	140
Number of REM periods	0.04	[−0.60, 0.67]	0.32	0.11	3.60	44.38	3	40	30
Slow-wave sleep duration	0.03	[−0.51, 0.57]	0.28	0.08	—	—	2	27	23
% slow-wave sleep	−0.07	[−0.42, 0.28]	0.18	0.03	22.53**	60.05	10	174	132
Stage 1 duration	0.25	[−0.36, 0.87]	0.31	0.10	—	—	2	19	19
Stage 2 duration	−0.68*	[−1.23, −0.12]	0.28	0.08	—	—	2	27	23
% stage 1 sleep	0.13	[−0.11, 0.36]	0.12	0.01	3.71	0.00	9	164	137
% stage 2 sleep	0.19	[−0.30, 0.67]	0.25	0.06	39.89**	77.44	10	190	153
% stage 3 sleep	0.31	[−0.38, 1.00]	0.35	0.12	10.43**	71.24	4	97	54
% stage 4 sleep	−0.31	[−1.10, 0.47]	0.40	0.16	13.28**	77.41	4	97	54

Note: Q = weighted sum of squares, indicates total dispersion; I^2 = proportion of variance due to real differences in effect size; PD = panic disorder; REM sleep = rapid eye movement sleep; slow-wave sleep = stages 3 and 4 sleep; — = insufficient number of studies to report heterogeneity; CI = confidence interval.
**= Significant differences between groups, $p < 0.05$.*
***= Significant heterogeneity, $p < 0.05$.*

Table 3.
Meta-analysis results for polysomnographic and actigraphic data.

reported NPA frequency: at least one lifetime NPA, one or more NPA in the past month, and two NPA per month or per 2 months with apprehensiveness about possible future NPA. For the latter criterion, the intensity of apprehensiveness about NPA had to be a minimum of four on a scale of 1–8. Finally, both NPA and

Frequency criteria	Event rate (prevalence %)	Confidence interval (95%)	Q	I^2	Number of studies	Sample size
1 or more lifetime NPA	52.1	[46.4, 57.7]	36.51*	75.34	10	1647
1 NPA in the last month	27.0	[17.9, 38.6]	8.47*	64.59	4	224
2 NPA/month or /2 months with apprehensiveness 4/8, lasting at least 6 months	40.9	[18.1, 68.5]	—	—	2	221

Note: Q = weighted sum of squares, indicates total dispersion; I^2 = proportion of variance due to real differences in effect size; PD = panic disorder; NPA = nocturnal panic attack; — = insufficient number of studies to report heterogeneity; CI = confidence interval.
**= Significant heterogeneity, $p < 0.05$.*

Table 4.
Meta-analysis results for NPA prevalence.

apprehensiveness had to be present for at least the prior 6 months. A meta-analysis was performed for each of the three categories, with frequency of NPA in patients with PD and PD group sample size as input data. Results indicated that, among the pooled sample of patients with PD, an average of 52.1% (95% CI [46.4, 57.7]) reported at least one lifetime NPA (**Table 4**). The heterogeneity test revealed significant heterogeneity between studies and indicated that 73% of observed variance was attributed to true effects. The prevalence rate of one or more NPA in the past month was 27.0% (95% CI [17.9, 38.6]), and the heterogeneity test was significant. Sixty-five percent of observed variance was attributed to true effects. For recurrent NPA (2/month or/2 months with apprehensiveness about possible future NPA, intensity of apprehensiveness of minimally four on a scale of 1–8.), the mean prevalence rate was 40.9% (95% CI [18.1, 68.5]). As analyses included only two studies, heterogeneity was not calculated.

4. Discussion

This study was designed to use meta-analytic methodology to draw a detailed portrait of sleep disturbances in PD. More specifically, the primary objective was to compare sleep in this population to sleep in healthy controls. Results from subjective and objective data analysis confirmed the hypothesis that sleep quality in the former group is significantly poorer than in the latter group. Furthermore, in comparison to controls, patients with PD take longer to fall asleep and have more sleep disturbances and more difficulty with daytime functioning secondary to sleep problems. Analysis of objective sleep data revealed differences between patients with PD and healthy controls in sleep continuity parameters: patients with PD take longer to fall asleep, have a shorter sleep duration, and demonstrate poorer sleep efficiency. For the majority of sleep architecture parameters, no differences were noted between patients with PD and control participants, with the exception of stage 2 duration, which was shorter in patients with PD.

4.1 Self-report data

To date, some literature reviews have explored subjective sleep complaints in PD [3, 38–40]. They reported conclusions that are consistent with the data reported here, indicating that patients with PD report significant subjective sleep alterations. However, most reviews did not detail the nature of these complaints. For example, Mellman [39] reported that there was subjective insomnia in patients with

PD, but without further specifying if there was a problem with sleep onset, sleep maintenance, or early awakenings. Only one recent systematic literature review has provided greater precision on subjective sleep complaints by reporting the results of nine previous studies in a structured manner [3]. This study reports a wide range of measures such as the sleep-wake experience list [45], the PSQI [18, 21, 46, 47], and the Goldberg depression and anxiety scales [48]. This unites useful and diverse information about the sleep of patients with PD. However, equivalence of measures and results synthesis remains difficult to judge. The statistical procedures of meta-analysis that we used allowed us to carry out the said synthesis and provided easily understandable summary indicators (size effects) of the results.

The elevated level of heterogeneity in PSQI global scores constitutes one critical point for consideration in our analysis of subjective sleep data. Variation in effect sizes is significant, and the majority of variance (92.8%) is attributable to differences in true effects. The observed elevated level of heterogeneity may be attributable to hidden covariates that moderate the differences between patients with PD and healthy controls. Previous research has identified subgroups of patients with PD in which insomnia might be more prevalent, including patients reporting NPA, depression [45], and greater anxiety sensitivity [18]. Effect sizes reported in each individual study may vary according to whether participants from these subgroups were included. Unfortunately, the number of studies reporting PSQI global scores was too low to permit the investigation of the impact of such variables via meta-regression [32]. Further research addressing the impact of covariates such as NPA, depression, and anxiety sensitivity on sleep quality in PD patients is warranted.

4.2 Objective data

Among objective sleep variables, previous literature reviews reported impairments in sleep continuity parameters. Reports of sleep onset latency, sleep efficiency, and total sleep time alterations were the most cited and robust [3, 39, 40]. Some authors also mentioned that patients with PD have difficulty maintaining sleep [39], with higher percentage of wake time [40]. Combined effect sizes from our findings indeed confirm that patients with PD have shorter sleep, take longer to fall asleep, and have poorer sleep efficiency. However, they do not confirm previous findings regarding sleep maintenance, since total wake time and number of awakenings were similar in PD and control groups. Based on these results, the nature of sleep difficulties in PD seems to be restricted to sleep onset and early awakenings, rather than sleep maintenance.

Previous reviews highlighted the existing inconsistencies in sleep architecture data. Overall, they report that there is as much evidence showing that the sleep architecture of patients with PD and of healthy controls is different as there is evidence that they are not [3, 40]. The narrative nature of previous reviews limited the conclusions that could be drawn from such data. Given this limit, the present study used meta-analysis to synthesize conflicting data. Results showed no difference between the sleep of patients with PD and the sleep of healthy control participants on the percentages of stage 1 and stage 2 sleep, of slow-wave sleep, and of REM sleep. Also, there were no differences between groups for the number of REM periods, REM sleep density and duration, stages 1 and 2 sleep duration, slow-wave sleep duration, and percentages of stage 3 and of stage 4 sleep. However, the latter results were less reliable due to the small number of studies that were included (two to four studies for each variable). Therefore, confirmation of the results is needed.

In sum, there is reliable evidence that, in comparison to healthy controls, patients with PD demonstrate alterations in objective sleep latency, sleep efficiency, and total sleep time. Also, it is plausible that percentages of REM sleep, of delta sleep, and of stage 1 and stage 2 sleep do not differ between patients with PD and controls. For other variables, further research is required to confirm existing results.

4.3 Why is sleep altered in PD?

A recent literature review highlighted the need for studies to go beyond mere descriptions of sleep disturbances and to investigate the role of sleep disturbances in the development and maintenance of PD [3]. Research on the impact of cognitive activity on sleep yielded important insights into the onset of insomnia in PD. Studies of the possible links between repetitive thought (e.g., worry or rumination) and various sleep characteristics in college students indicated that repetitive thoughts impact sleep [49]. Since patients with PD often worry about having panic attacks, it is possible that reported sleep alterations could be associated with repetitive worry about future panic. This hypothesis is consistent with Harvey's [14] cognitive model of insomnia, which proposes that excess negative cognitive activity plays a central role in the maintenance of insomnia.

In patients with PD, the content of repetitive thinking often relates to possible panic attacks and their consequences. Patients develop a fear of anxiety itself, i.e., anxiety sensitivity [18, 50]. Researchers have found that, in patients with PD, anxiety sensitivity is linked to insomnia and, in particular, to longer sleep latency [18]. Authors hypothesized that anxiety sensitivity makes patients monitor their anxiety signs and symptoms and could increase levels of cognitive, emotional, and physiological activation [18]. This state of activation could disrupt the healthy course of sleep [18].

Sleep impairment caused by activation could be the beginning of a cycle where anxiety and insomnia mutually feed each other. Evidence suggests that sleep deprivation induces activation and anxiety in the general population [12] and increases the risk of panic in patients with PD [13]. Therefore, it is hypothesized that a sleep deficit could increase the risk of panic by inducing activation and anxiety. Indeed, since patients with PD fear signs of anxiety, the activation and anxiety caused by the sleep deficit trigger more anxiety that can culminate into panic attacks. These panic attacks could further disrupt sleep because of the activation state they caused and apprehensiveness. Future research should aim at verifying the hypothesis of the vicious cycle between panic and insomnia in order to better understand the cognitive, behavioral, and emotional mechanisms behind the sleep disturbances identified in the present study.

The majority of the results issued from objective data were consistent with cognitive models of insomnia and PD. In contrast, the finding that patients with PD have shorter stage 2 sleep is not intuitive. One possible explanation for this result is the inclusion of patients with NPA. Since NPA usually occur between stage 2 and stage 3 sleep, there may be a relationship between the presence of NPA and decreased stage 2 sleep. An alternative explanation is that shorter stage 2 sleep is an artifact of overall shorter sleep time. Since stage 2 sleep is the longest stage over the course of a night's sleep (i.e., 45–55% of total sleep time; [51]), the changes in sleep continuity observed in our study (longer sleep latency, lower sleep efficiency, and shorter total sleep time) may be attributable to shorter sleep in all three stages. Since stage 2 occupies the majority of the night, it may be the only stage for which the change can be statistically detected. Indeed, the fact that the percentage of stage 2 sleep observed in patients with PD does not differ significantly from that observed in control subjects supports this hypothesis.

Gathering detailed data on the nature of subjective and objective insomnia is a first step toward a greater understanding of the mechanisms (e.g., cognitions, anxiety sensitivity, repetitive thinking, etc.) through which insomnia could maintain panic symptoms and vice versa. Nevertheless, the present review does not permit further inferences about interactions between sleep and PD. Considering that analyses of PSQI component scales, stages 1 and 2 sleep duration, slow-wave sleep (duration of slow-wave sleep, percentage of stages 3 and 4), and REM sleep (duration, density, number of REM periods) are based on a small number of studies (between two and four), further research is required to confirm the specific nature of sleep alterations, particularly regarding sleep architecture.

4.4 Nocturnal panic attacks

This study's secondary aim was to estimate the prevalence rate of NPA. Results indicated that, among patients with PD, 52.1% (95% CI [46.4, 57.7]) experienced at least one lifetime NPA and 27.0% (95% CI [17.9, 38.6]) experienced at least one panic attack in the past month. Furthermore, 40.9% (95% CI [18.1, 68.5]) of patients with PD reported recurrent NPA (at least 1–2/month in the past 6 months) with apprehensiveness about possible future nocturnal attacks. Of the three estimates, the lifetime prevalence obtained here is the most precise and reliable, with a confidence interval ranging from 46.4 to 57.7%. This represents an improvement compared to previously reported estimates: 44–71% in Lee and Douglass [38], 18–69% in Mellman [39], and 33–71% in Papadimitriou and Linkowski [40]. The two other NPA prevalence estimates calculated in our meta-analysis have wider confidence intervals, indicating poorer reliability. The poorer reliability may explain why the prevalence rate is higher using a more restrictive criterion (1/month or/2 months, with apprehensiveness, present since 6 months; 40.9%) than using a less restrictive criterion (one NPA in the past month; 27.0%). These results may be attributable to measurement error rather than to real differences in prevalence.

Some authors have proposed that NPA could be linked to abnormalities in breathing regulation and patterns [52]. Previous research has suggested that patients with PD have chronic hyperventilation [53], which would cause CO_2 depletion in the blood [54]. The metabolism would then adapt and become more sensitive to small increases of CO_2 in the blood [52]. Since non-REM sleep stages imply a reduced breathing rate and, therefore, a rise in CO_2, authors propose that they could be sufficient to induce the physiological reactions and physical sensations that are feared by people with PD [54, 55]. Considering that there have been reports linking nocturnal panic to sleep apnea [56], we could hypothesize that sleep apnea could induce even stronger physiological sensations in people with CO_2 hypersensitivity. Therefore, they would be more at risk of having NPA. However, the abnormalities in breathing regulation cannot totally explain the presence of NPA. Cognitive components such as beliefs about physiological sensations and interoceptive conditioning still have to be present in order for NPA to occur.

4.5 Limitations

Interpretation of the present findings should take into account the following limitations. Some variables were reported by very few studies. For example, only two studies reported data on PSQI subscales, slow-wave sleep, and stage 1 and stage 2 sleep duration. On the one hand, the limited data increases the risk of biased results, as there is no guarantee that the two included effect sizes are representative of the entire distribution of true effects [32]. On the other hand, a risk inherent to not running the analyses also exists, as it allows for the possibility of vote-counting, which is even more biased [32]. For example, Papadimitriou and Linkowski [40] discussed conflicting results about self-reported sleep efficiency. With only results of individual studies available, the authors could not draw concrete conclusions.

Our meta-analysis did not provide a clear conclusion either, but allowed us to contribute to the knowledge in this area by statistically synthesizing the data, taking into consideration the relative weight of each study, and providing a confidence interval for a true effect.

A significant number of studies with subjective sleep data could not be used because they used diverse self-report questionnaires. For example, a study by Batterham et al. in 2012 [48] was the only one to use the Goldberg depression and anxiety scale questions about sleep. While some of the data could have been merged into a single analysis designed to answer the question "Is there a significant difference in subjective sleep between patients with PD and healthy controls?", such an analysis would not have provided information about specific sleep disturbances.

The majority of studies using PSQI did not report scores for the seven subscales. The inclusion of this data would have permitted a better comparison of subjective and objective sleep data. Previous research indicates that there is a misperception of sleep in some subjects with insomnia, who overestimate sleep onset latency and underestimate total sleep time [57, 58]. Conversely, other subjects tend to overestimate their total sleep time [58]. It would have been interesting to compare the results of the meta-analysis for subjective and objective sleep data. Future research should emphasize precision in reports of subjective sleep complaints.

The absence of standards in NPA reporting complicated study comparison, with the result that many studies were excluded from our estimates. Moreover, few authors specified whether or not apprehensiveness about possible future NPA was present. As discussed previously, the presence of apprehensiveness is important because it is hypothesized to increase arousal and maintain insomnia. In the absence of apprehensiveness, interactions between NPA, insomnia, and PD are less clear. We therefore suggest the use of standardized frequency criteria for NPA prevalence that include apprehensiveness about future NPA. The criterion used by Craske et al. [59] and Albert et al. [60] constitutes a good example. The use of a standardized measure of NPA (e.g., the appendix to ADIS-IV for NPA) would contribute to the generation of standardized data. This section of the ADIS-IV is clinician-administered; developing a self-report version could also make standardized evaluation of NPA more accessible. However, since ADIS-IV has been updated to ADIS-5, an update of the appendix to DSM-5 criteria is needed before any other developments take place.

5. Conclusion

In conclusion, this systematic literature review confirms the presence of both subjective and objective insomnia in patients with PD. The results indicate that sporadic NPA are common in this population, i.e., more than one in every two patients with PD (52.1%) report at least one lifetime NPA. Recurrent NPA with apprehensiveness about future episodes seems to be slightly less common (40.9%) and is hypothesized to trigger and maintain insomnia. However the reliability of this last prevalence is low and needs confirming in future research.

We would like to emphasize the importance of using standardized psychometric tools such as the PSQI when reporting research data about sleep in patients with PD. Moreover, reporting results for subscales could give a better and more complete idea of the type of sleep alterations patients are experiencing. Also, research in this area would benefit from greater standardization in reports of subjective sleep and NP, and from particular attention in detailing subscales and information about diverse sleep variables (e.g., sleep latency, sleep efficiency, awakenings, etc.).

Finally, we would like to highlight the need for new research reporting polysomnographic data from patients with PD. Indeed, many of the studies included in our review were completed over 20 years ago. With the publication of DSM-5, the need for current data is even greater. Such studies could also be designed to help understand the cognitive processes by which insomnia is generated and maintained. Polysomnographic studies could also help understand the role of sleep-disordered breathing in NPA. Further study of sleep in patients with PD is particularly important because sleep problems are associated with poorer outcomes in individuals presenting psychopathology [61, 62]. Given the link between PD and sleep disturbances, such research could yield significant benefits for clinical evaluation and treatment of patients with PD.

Conflict of interest

The authors have no conflict of interest to declare.

Author details

Geneviève Belleville* and Alenka Potočnik
School of Psychology, Laval University, Quebec City, Canada

*Address all correspondence to: genevieve.belleville@psy.ulaval.ca

References

[1] Kessler RC, Chiu WT, Jin R, Ruscio AM, Shear K, Walters EE. The epidemiology of panic attacks, panic disorder, and agoraphobia in the National Comorbidity Survey Replication. Archives of General Psychiatry. 2006;**63**(4):415-424

[2] American Psychiatric Association. Diagnostic and Statistical Manual of Mental Disorders (DSM-5). 5th ed. Washington, DC: American Psychiatric Publishing; 2013

[3] Cox RC, Olatunji BO. A systematic review of sleep disturbance in anxiety and related disorders. Journal of Anxiety Disorders. 2016;**37**:104-129

[4] American Psychiatric Association. Diagnostic and Statistical Manual of Mental Disorders, Text Rev. 4th ed. Washington, DC: Author; 2000

[5] Buysse DJ, Ancoli-Israel S, Edinger JD, Lichstein KL, Morin CM. Recommendations for a standard research assessment of insomnia. Sleep. 2006;**29**(9):1155-1173

[6] Hauri PJ, Friedman M, Ravaris CL. Sleep in patients with spontaneous panic attacks. Sleep. 1989;**12**(4):323-337

[7] Nakamura M, Sugiura T, Nidhida S, Komada Y, Inoue Y. Is nocturnal panic a distinct disease category? Comparison of clinical characteristics among patients with primary nocturnal panic, daytime panic, and coexistence of nocturnal and daytime panic. Journal of Clinical Sleep Medicine. 2013;**9**(5):461-467

[8] Rosenfeld DS, Furman Y. Pure sleep panic: Two case reports and a review of the literature. Sleep. 1994;**17**(5):462-465

[9] Pattyn T, Van Den Eede F, Lamers F, Veltman D, Sabbe BG, Penninx BW. Identifying panic disorder subtypes using factor mixture modeling. Depression and Anxiety. 2015;**32**(7):509-517

[10] Agargun MY, Kara H. Recurrent sleep panic, insomnia, and suicidal behavior in patients with panic disorder. Comprehensive Psychiatry. 1998;**39**(3):149-151

[11] Uhde TW. The anxiety disorders. In: Kryger MH, Roth T, Dement WC, editors. Principles and Practice of Sleep Medicine. 2nd ed. Philadelphia: WB Saunders; 1994. pp. 871-898

[12] Babson KA, Feldner MT, Trainor CD, Smith RC. An experimental investigation of the effects of acute sleep deprivation on panic-relevant biological challenge responding. Behavior Therapy. 2009;**40**(3):239-250

[13] Roy-Byrne PP, Uhde TW, Post RM. Effects of one night's sleep deprivation on mood and behavior in panic disorder: Patients with panic disorder compared with depressed patients and normal controls. Archives of General Psychiatry. 1986;**43**:895-899

[14] Harvey AG. A cognitive model of insomnia. Behaviour Research and Therapy. 2002;**40**(8):869-894

[15] Craske MG, Barlow DH. Panic disorder and agoraphobia. In: Barlow DH, editor. Clinical Handbook of Psychological Disorders: A Step-by-Step Treatment Manual. 5th ed. New York, NY, US: Guilford Press; 2014. pp. 1-61

[16] Adler CM, Craske MG, Barlow DH. Relaxation-induced panic (RIP): When resting isn't peaceful. Integrative Psychiatry. 1987;**5**(2):94-100

[17] Aikins DE, Craske MG. Sleep-based heart period variability in panic disorder with and without nocturnal panic

attacks. Journal of Anxiety Disorders. 2008;**22**(3):453-463

[18] Hoge EA, Marques L, Wechsler RS, Lasky AK, Delong HR, Jacoby RJ, et al. The role of anxiety sensitivity in sleep disturbance in panic disorder. Journal of Anxiety Disorders. 2011;**25**(4):536-538

[19] Saletu-Zyhlarz GM, Anderer PA, Berger P, Gruber G, Oberndorfer S, Saletu B. Nonorganic insomnia in panic disorder: Comparative sleep laboratory studies with normal controls and placebo-controlled trials with alprazolam. Human Psychopharmacology: Clinical and Experimental. 2000;**15**:241-254

[20] Stein MB, Chartier M, Walker JR. Sleep in nondepressed patients with panic disorder: I. systematic assessment of subjective sleep quality and sleep disturbance. Sleep. 1993;**16**(8):724-726

[21] Todder D, Baune BT. Quality of sleep in escitalopram-treated female patients with panic disorder. Human Psychopharmacology: Clinical and Experimental. 2010;**25**(2):167-173

[22] Mellman TA, Uhde TW. Electroencephalographic sleep in panic disorder: A focus on sleep-related panic attacks. Archives of General Psychiatry. 1989;**46**(2):178-184

[23] Arriaga F, Lara E, Matos-Pires A, Cavaglia F, Bastos L. Diagnostic relevance of sleep complaints in anxiety and mood disorders. European Psychiatry. 1995;**10**(8):386-390

[24] Hranov LG. Sleep disorders and nocturnal panic attacks in panic disorder. Journal of Sleep Research. 2002;**11**(Suppl. 1):109

[25] Okasha A, Bishry Z, Khalil AH, Darwish TA, el Dawla AS, Shohdy A. Panic disorder: An overlapping or independent entity? The British Journal of Psychiatry. 1994;**164**(6):818-825

[26] Arriaga F, Paiva T, Matos-Pires A, Cavaglia F, Lara E, Bastos L. The sleep of non-depressed patients with panic disorder: A comparison with normal controls. Acta Psychiatrica Scandinavica. 1996;**93**:191-194

[27] Uhde TW, Roy-Byrne P, Gillin JC, Mendelson WB, Boulenger JP, Vittone BJ, et al. The sleep of patients with panic disorder: A preliminary report. Psychiatry Research. 1984;**12**(3):251-259

[28] Stein MB, Enns MW, Kryger MH. Sleep in nondepressed patients with panic disorder: II. Polysomnographic assessment of sleep architecture and sleep continuity. Journal of Affective Disorders. 1993;**28**(1):1-6

[29] Lydiard RB, Zealberg J, Laraia MT, Fossey M, Prockow V, Gross J, et al. Electroencephalography during sleep of patients with panic disorder. The Journal of Neuropsychiatry and Clinical Neurosciences. 1989;**1**:372-376

[30] Lauer CJ, Krieg J-C, Garcia-Borreguero D, Özdaglar A, Holsboer F. Panic disorder and major depression: A comparative electroencephalographic sleep study. Psychiatry Research. 1992;**44**:41-54

[31] Canetti A, de la Fuente JR, Salin-Pascual R, Gutierrez R. Características del sueño en pacientes con crisis de angustia [Sleep characteristics of patients with panic attacks]. Acta Psiquiátrica y Psicológica de América Latina. 1987;**33**(1):21-26

[32] Borenstein M, Hedges LV, Higgins JPT, Rothstein HR, editors. Introduction to Meta-Analysis. Chichester, United Kingdom: John Wiley and Sons; 2009

[33] Schredl M, Kronenberg G, Nonnell P, Heuser I. Dream recall, nightmare frequency, and nocturnal panic attacks in patients with panic disorder. The

Journal of Nervous and Mental Disease. 2001;**189**(8):559-562

[34] Pirildar S, Bayraktar E, Berdeli A, Kucuk O, Alkin T, Kose T. Progesterone receptor gene polymorphism in panic disorder: Associations with agoraphobia and respiratory subtype of panic disorder. Bulletin of Clinical Psychopharmacology. 2010;**20**(2):153-159

[35] Freed S, Craske MG, Greher MR. Nocturnal panic and trauma. Depression and Anxiety. 1999;**9**(3):141-145

[36] Labbate LA, Pollack MH, Otto MW, Langenauer S, Rosenbaum JF. Sleep panic attacks: An association with childhood anxiety and adult psychopathology. Biological Psychiatry. 1994;**36**(1):57-60

[37] Agargun MY, Kara H. Sleep panic attacks in patients with panic disorder: The association with major depression. European Psychiatry. 1997;**12**:42-43

[38] Lee EK, Douglass AB. Sleep in psychiatric disorders: Where are we now? The Canadian Journal of Psychiatry. 2010;**55**(7):403-412

[39] Mellman TA. Sleep and anxiety disorders. Sleep Medicine Clinics. 2008;**3**(2):261-268

[40] Papadimitriou GN, Linkowski P. Sleep disturbance in anxiety disorders. International Review of Psychiatry. 2005;**17**(4):229-236

[41] Meritt-Davis O, Balon R. Nocturnal panic: Biology, psychopathology, and its contribution to the expression of panic disorder. Depression and Anxiety. 2003;**18**:221-227

[42] Moher D, Liberati A, Tetzlaff J, Altman DG, The PRISMA Group. Preferred reporting items for systematic reviews and meta-analyses: The PRISMA statement. PLoS Medicine. 2009;**6**(7)

[43] Conn VS, Valentine JC, Cooper HM, Rantz MJ. Grey literature in meta-analyses. Nursing Research. 2003;**52**(4):256-261

[44] Cohen J. A power primer. Psychological Bulletin. 1992;**122**:155-159

[45] Overbeek T, van Diest R, Schruers K, Kruizinga F, Griez E. Sleep complaints in panic disorder patients. The Journal of Nervous and Mental Disease. 2005;**193**(7):488-493

[46] Swinkels CM, Ulmer CS, Beckham JC, Buse N, Calhoun PS. The association of sleep duration, mental health, and health risk behaviors among U.S. Afghanistan/Iraq era veterans. Sleep. 2013;**36**(7):1019-1025

[47] Ramsawh HJ, Weisberg RB, Dyck I, Stout R, Keller MB. Age of onset, clinical characteristics, and 15-year course of anxiety disorders in a prospective, longitudinal, observational study. Journal of Affective Disorders. 2011;**132**(1-2):260-264

[48] Batterham PJ, Glozier N, Christensen H. Sleep disturbance, personality and the onset of depression and anxiety: Prospective cohort study. The Australian and New Zealand Journal of Psychiatry. 2012;**46**(11):1089-1098

[49] Takano K, Sakamoto S, Tanno Y. Repetitive thought impairs sleep quality: An experience sampling study. Behavior Therapy. 2014;**45**:67-82

[50] Reiss S, Peterson RA, Gursky DM, McNally RJ. Anxiety sensitivity, anxiety frequency and the predictions of fearfulness. Behaviour Research and Therapy. 1986;**24**(1):1-8

[51] Carskadon MA, Dement WC. Normal human sleep: An overview.

In: Kryger MH, Roth T, Dement WC, editors. Principles and Practice of Sleep Medicine. Philadelphia, PA: Elsevier; 2011. pp. 16-25

[52] Ley R. Panic attacks during sleep: A hyperventilation-probability model. Journal of Behavior Therapy and Experimental Psychiatry. 1988;**19**(3):181-192

[53] Grassi M, Caldirola D, Vanni G, Guerriero G, Piccinni M, Valchera A, et al. Baseline respiratory parameters in panic disorder: A meta-analysis. Journal of Affective Disorders. 2013;**146**(2):158-173

[54] Craske MG, Rowe M. Nocturnal panic. Clinical Psychology: Science and Practice. 1997;**4**(2):153-174

[55] Gorman J, Fyer MR, Goetz R, Askanazi J, Liebowitz MR, Fyer A, et al. Ventilatory physiology of patients with panic disorder. Archives of General Psychiatry. 1988;**45**:31-39

[56] Edlund MJ, McNamara ME, Millman RP. Sleep apnea and panic attacks. Comprehensive Psychiatry. 1991;**32**(2):130-132

[57] Harvey AG, Tang NKY. (Mis) perception of sleep in insomnia: A puzzle and a resolution. Psychological Bulletin. 2012;**138**(1):77-101

[58] Fernandez-Mendoza J, Calhoun SL, Bixler EO, Karataraki M, Liao D, Vela-Bueno A, et al. Sleep misperception and chronic insomnia in the general population: Role of objective sleep duration and psychological profiles. Psychosomatic Medicine. 2011;**73**(1):88-97

[59] Craske MG, Golinelli D, Stein MB, Roy-Byrne P, Bystritsky A, Sherbourne C. Does the addition of cognitive behavioral therapy improve panic disorder treatment outcome relative to medication alone in the primary-care setting? Psychological Medicine. 2005;**35**(11):1645-1654

[60] Albert U, Maina G, Bergesio C, Bogetto F. Axis I and II comorbidities in subjects with and without nocturnal panic. Depression and Anxiety. 2006;**23**(7):422-428

[61] Ohayon MM, Roth T. Place of chronic insomnia in the course of depressive and anxiety disorders. Journal of Psychiatric Research. 2003;**37**(1):9-15

[62] van Mill JG, Vogelzangs N, van Someren EJW, Hoogendijk WJG, Penninx BWJH. Sleep duration, but not insomnia, predicts the 2-year course of depressive and anxiety disorders. The Journal of Clinical Psychiatry. 2014;**75**(2):119-126

Chapter 8

Panic Attacks and Panic Disorder

Dimitar Bonevski and Andromahi Naumovska

Abstract

A panic attack is an intense wave of fear characterized by its unexpectedness and debilitating, immobilizing intensity. Regardless of the cause, panic attacks are treatable. The signs and symptoms of a panic attack develop abruptly and usually reach their peak within 10 min. Panic attack symptoms may include hyperventilation, heart racing, chest pain, and trembling, sweating, and dizziness, with a fear of losing control, going crazy, or dying. Although the exact causes of panic attacks and panic disorder are unclear, the tendency to have panic attacks runs in families. There also appears to be a connection with major life transitions and severe stress. Treatment for panic attacks and panic disorder include psychotherapy and medication.

Keywords: panic attacks, panic disorder, symptoms, causes, treatment

1. Introduction

A panic attack is an intensive fear characterized by unexpectedness and immobilizing intensity. Often strikes without any warning, very often with no clear trigger, and also may occur when the person is relaxed or even when is asleep. Panic attacks are common. A panic attack can be a one-time occurrence, but usually many people experience repeat episodes, in a longer lifetime period. Among persons that ever had a PA, the majority had recurrent PAs (66.5, s.e. 0.5%). Most people recover without treatment, only a few of them from panic attacks develop panic disorder. Lifetime prevalence of PAs is 13.2% (s.e. 0.1%) [18].

Sometimes recurrent panic attacks are often triggered by a specific situation, in which the person felt endangered before. A panic attack may also occur as part of another disorder, such as panic disorder, social phobia, or depression.

Depending on the relationship between the occurrence of the attack and absence or presence of situational triggers, panic attacks can be divided into the following:

- Unexpected (untested) panic attacks in which the occurrence of a panic attack is not related to a situation trigger (occurs spontaneously as a lightning strike) and is the most common type of attack in the PD [44].

- Situational-induced (triggered) panic attacks, which almost invariably occur immediately after exposure, or the anticipation of a trigger situation (e.g., seeing a snake or dog always triggers an immediate panic attack).

- Situational predisposed panic attacks, which is highly expected to occur when exposed to the trigger situation but are not inseparably linked to the trigger, and it is not necessary to occur immediately after exposure (e.g., panic attacks

IntechOpen

are more likely to occur during the ride, but sometimes individuals they can drive and have no panic attacks, or they happen half an hour after the ride).

- Other types of attacks are those that occur in a special emotional context those involving limited symptoms as well night attacks.

- Situational-induced attacks are more characteristic of social and specific phobias. Situationally predisposed panic attacks are particularly common in panic disorder, but can also occur in specific and social phobias.

The onset of unexpected panic attacks is necessary for the diagnosis of panic disorder with or without agoraphobia.

The frequency and severity of panic attacks vary widely. For example, some individuals have intermediate frequency attacks (e.g., once a week), which occur constantly for months. Others report frequent attacks in a short period (day, week) that are separated for a long period (weeks or months) without seizures or with rare attacks (two per month) over a long period of time. Attacks with limited symptoms (e.g., identical to full panic attacks, but with fewer associated symptoms) are very common in panic disorder.

2. Manifestation and diagnosis of panic disorder

2.1 The signs and symptoms of a panic attack

The signs and symptoms of a panic attack may include hyperventilation, heart racing, chest pain, and trembling, sweating, and dizziness, with a fear of losing control, going crazy, or dying.

2.2 The signs and symptoms of panic disorder

Among persons that ever had a PA only 12.8% fulfilled DSM-5 criteria for PD. In comparison with panic attacks, panic disorder is characterized by repeated panic attacks. Panic disorder (PD) is a chronic mental disorder with essential features such as recurrent panic attacks, persisting concern about the attacks, and a change in behavior as a result of the attacks [17].

The lifetime prevalence of PD is two times more likely to occur in women than in men [32]. Age of onset for PD is a wide range between 25 and 53 years regardless of gender. Alongside the variation in age, the most probable period is the late adolescence and the middle of the 1930s. A certain number of PD cases begin in childhood or after 45 years of age [33]. Panic disorder usually begins in late adolescence or early adulthood and affects women about two times more often than men. The median age of onset is 32. Cross-national lifetime prevalence estimates is 1.7% for PD [18].

Individuals with PD show distinctive concern about the consequences of panic attacks. Some fear that attacks indicate the presence of an undetected life-threatening disease (e.g., heart disease), and others fear that panic attacks indicate that they are causing, losing control, or being emotionally weak. However, patients with PD do not necessarily show deterioration in the quality of their lives by becoming prisoners of panic attacks [17]. Some individuals with PD significantly change their behavior (e.g., they leave work). Concerns about the next attack or its consequences are often associated with avoiding behavior. Hence, PD is defined as an experience of having panic attacks and as emotional and behavioral consequences from it.

2.3 Diagnosis of panic disorder

To help pinpoint a diagnosis it is necessary to do:

- Complete physical exam.
- Blood tests to check the thyroid and other possible conditions and tests on heart, such as an electrocardiogram (ECG or EKG).
- Psychological evaluation about symptoms, fears or concerns, stressful situations, relationship problems, situations that are avoided, and family history. Fill out a psychological self-assessment or questionnaire.
- Check alcohol or other substance use.

Criteria for diagnosis of panic disorder according to ICD-10 are:

- At least 1 month many attacks with vegetative anxiety which occur in circumstances where there is no objective danger;
- Panic attacks are without restrictions on known and predictable situations
- There is no symptoms of anxiety between seizures (although anxiety may be common)
- Psychological or vegetative symptoms are primary manifestations of anxiety, and not secondary to other symptoms, such as crazy ideas or obsessive thoughts;
- Anxiety must be limited to at least two of the following situations (or mainly to occur only in them): crowds, public places, travel from home, or unaccompanied travel by another person;
- Avoiding the phobic situation

A single panic attack may only last a few minutes, up to 20–30 min, but can cause serious problems in the everyday life. This can also lead to:

- Anticipatory anxiety in between panic attacks, the patient feels anxiety and tension, because of a fear of having future panic attacks. This "fear of fear" is present most of the time, and can be extremely disabling in everyday life.
- Phobic avoidance of certain situations or environments. This avoidance may be based on the belief that the situation that is avoided caused the previous panic attack, or is a place where the escape is difficult or the help is unavailable in case of a panic attack. Taken to its extreme, phobic avoidance becomes agoraphobia.

3. Causes of panic attacks and panic disorder

The causes have not been fully illuminated, although there are a number of theories.

3.1 Biological theories and pathophysiology of panic attacks and panic disorder

From biological theories, there is a genetic predisposition and disturbance in the functioning of certain neurotransmitter systems in the brain (noradrenergic, serotonergic, dopaminergic, GABA). During panic attack an excessive vegetative reaction, with an increased tonus of sympathetic system is present, and also with increased catecholamine release [20].

The exact pathophysiology of PD is currently unknown. There are theories that functioning of serotonin, norepinephrine, dopamine and gamma-aminobutyric acid (GABA) neurotransmitter systems play a role [42].

- The noradrenergic theory assumes that in PD presynaptic norepinephrine auto-receptors are hypersensitive to stimulation by norepinephrine [31].

- Other clinical studies demonstrate that medications increasing the synaptic availability of 5-HT, are effective in the treatment of PD. Rival theories of 5-HT deficiency vs. excess attempt to explain the impact of 5-HT function in PD [41].

- Researches are indicating that GABA may play a role—PD is a result of a lack of central inhibition and decreased GABA concentrations, leading to uncontrolled anxiety during panic attacks [24, 26].

3.2 Psychological theories

As a special predisposing characteristic of people who are prone to the development of panic disorder, the existence of anxiety character is emphasized, which is manifest in childhood as a tendency to shame, cold and wet palms, fear of illness, constant need for support, hypersensitivity to the opinions of others, constant fear not to commit mistake, incompetence to accept responsibility, tranquility, scrupulousness, too high expectations of oneself.

Psychological theories speak of separation fears, the austerity of the release of sexual energy, the traumatized trauma, various misconceptions, or irrational thoughts, etc.

- Psychodynamic theory of panic attacks describes a state of regression in which a complete collapse of the defense defeats, anxiety overwhelms the person and is "empty" through panic states.

- Behavioral theory stresses that anxiety can be learned through the identification of the parent behavior model, then anxiety that develops after experiencing frightening stimuli, such as accidents, that are transmitted to other stimuli, as well as anxiety due to frustration that becomes a conditioned response to other stressful situations.

3.3 Researches: causes for panic attack and panic disorder

3.3.1 Genetic

Several studies have shown that the risk of PD is eight times higher in those with first-degree relatives with PD compared to those with no family history [40, 55]. Recent studies examine twins and estimate that the heritability of panic disorder is 30–40%.

A review of family and twin studies shows the highly familial nature of panic disorder and suggests evidence for a genetic etiology. The population-based lifetime rates of panic disorder cross-nationally range between 1.2/100 and 2.4/100, whereas, the lifetime rates in first-degree relatives of panic probands range between 7.7/100 and 20.5/100 [66].

3.3.2 Environmental

Combination of genetic and environment interactions can produce panic disorder [60]. Major stress and temperament that is more sensitive to stress or prone to negative emotions are connected with a onset of PD including major life transitions such (graduating from college and entering the workplace, getting married, or having a baby), and other severe stress (death of a loved one, divorce, or job loss) [21]. The aversive childhood events such as physical or sexual abuse have been associated with an increased risk of PD in adulthood [9, 10, 25].

3.3.3 Other

Asthma and smoking also have been associated with an increased risk of PD [13, 28]. Panic attacks can also be caused by medical conditions and other physical causes like mitral valve prolapse or hyperthyroidism [2, 34]. Substance abuse, especially stimulants (amphetamines, cocaine, and caffeine), may also be connected with the onset of panic attacks and PD.

4. Complications of panic attacks and panic disorder

Complications that panic attacks and panic disorders may cause avoidance of social situations, problems at work or school, depression with suicidal thoughts, substance abuse.

5. Treatment for panic disorder

The first contact of patient with PD usually is with a family physician. Due to the presence of numerous physical symptoms of panic attack, many people initially perform different somatic tests, from routine, to more complex, to internal and neurological examinations, and fail to timely initiate treatment. This is why the role of a family physician is important in recognizing and treating the disorder, or referring to a psychiatrist. Unfortunately only a minority of patients with panic disorder receive adequate care. One of the reasons is that about 50% of patients seek help [27, 36, 43].

Treatment of panic disorder should in no way be limited to providing first aid during panic attacks (usually by injection of diazepam intramuscularly as an emergency) without planning a targeted and ongoing treatment. The main treatment options are psychotherapy and medications. Combination of them is considered as the most effective [3].

5.1 Psychotherapy

Psychotherapy can help to understand panic attacks and panic disorder and learn how to cope with them.

- Individual therapy: That is, the most usual form of psychotherapy when dealing with panic disorder, but also other form of psychotherapy can be applied.

- Group therapy: Group therapy has positive sides because by sharing the experiences with others, people are creating opportunities for reinforcement by the others and decreasing their shame.

- Couples and family therapy: Symptoms of panic disorder usually affect the relations among the members in the family. Family and couple therapy helps them to improve the communication and to support the person with panic attack or disorder in an appropriate way.

5.1.1 Psychoanalysis and psychodynamic therapy

Psychoanalysis and psychodynamic therapy deals with problematic behavior, feeling, or thought by finding their unconscious meaning. When focused on panic deal with core conflicts in the person which are involving aggression and fearful dependency, or other intrapsychic conflicts that can also contribute to panic symptomatology [45].

5.1.2 Cognitive behavioral therapy

Cognitive-behavioral therapy involves teaching patients to recognize their distorted thinking. The goal is to clarify the patient's misinterpretation of the physical symptoms of panic attack and act on avoiding behavior by gradually exposing the situations that led to the attack. Useful relaxation exercises as well as regular breathing exercises, with moderate physical activity, are also useful.

In cognitive-behavioral treatment of panic disorder patients learn useful information about how and why anxiety, fear and panic occur, learn to apply various relaxation techniques, go through a gradual exposure to situations that create fear when are prepared, learn how their thoughts, assumptions and beliefs about anxiety and panic and their consequences worsen their problem and how they can deal with them, along with the therapy they go through various experiments to test their beliefs about fear and panic, and find out what to do in case of panic attacks [14].

Research shows that CBT efficacy is between 85 and 90% for treatment consisting of 12–15 meetings. In addition, most of the participants maintained this progress a year after treatment when monitored. Some studies have shown that CBT is at least as successful in the treatment of panic disorder as pharmacotherapy, but that treatment has been more prolonged by CBT. Namely, in CBT, an individual learns strategies to efficiently cope with his anxiety that is the skill he can use for his entire life [1, 49, 51, 67].

5.1.3 Humanistic therapy

Humanistic therapy (client-centered therapy, gestalt therapy, and existential therapy) is focused on people's capacities to make rational choices to use their potential and to accept the responsibility for themselves. It helps people to understand what is happening with them and to focus on the present by making new, more functional choices [65].

5.1.4 Self-help tips for panic attacks

The following self-help techniques can make a difference to overcome panic:

- Learn about panic and anxiety.
- Learn how to control your breathing. Deep breathing can relieve the symptoms of panic.
- Practice relaxation techniques—yoga, meditation, muscle relaxation to increase feelings of joy and equanimity.
- Exercise regularly. At least 30 min on most days (three 10-min sessions is just as good) like walking, running, swimming, or dancing can be especially effective.
- Connect face-to-face with family and friends. Symptoms of anxiety can become worse when you feel isolated, so building supportive friendships can help.
- Avoid smoking, alcohol, and caffeine.
- Get enough restful sleep [4].

5.2 Pharmacotherapy

There are a large number of drugs that have been studied in patients with panic disorder, but no drug has proven superior to other drugs used in the treatment of patients with panic disorder. Pharmacological agents with sufficient evidence to support their use in the treatment of panic disorder include:

- Antidepressants—selective serotonin reuptake inhibitors (SSRIs), serotonin noradrenaline reuptake inhibitor (SNRI), tricyclic antidepressants (TCAs) and
- Benzodiazepines [8, 37].

5.2.1 Antidepressants

The modern treatment of panic disorder is based on the use of antidepressants from the selective serotonin reuptake inhibitor (SSRI) and antidepressants from the serotonin and noradrenaline reuptake inhibitor (SNRI). Use of these drugs has less danger of creating addiction and abuse than benzodiazepines. The disadvantage of these antidepressants is delayed by the onset of the positive effect and adverse effects that occur during treatment.

Clinical studies have demonstrated the significant efficacy of SSRI/SNRI drugs in the treatment of panic disorder. Certain differences in medication do not occur in terms of efficacy, but can be observed in terms of side effects, drug delivery methods during their use, and the occurrence of deterioration in dose reduction and upon discontinuation of the drug. Therefore, it is important to pay attention to these factors in the individual selection of medicines. The dosage of antidepressants effective in panic disorder is shown in **Table 1**.

5.2.1.1 Efficacy of antidepressants in acute phase treatment of panic disorder

Antidepressants acting on the serotonergic system—citalopram, fluvoxamine, fluoxetine, paroxetine, sertraline [8, 16, 46, 61], the SNRIs venlafaxine and duloxetine [15, 35, 38, 58], and the TCAs imipramine and clomipramine [5, 39] are effective in treating acute phase of panic disorder.

Drug name	Start	Recommended	Maximum
Antidepressants SSRIs (mg/day)			
Citalopram	10	20–40	40
Escitalopram	5	10–20	20
Fluoxetine	10	20–40	60
Paroxetine	10	20–40	60
Sertraline	50	50–100	150
SNRIs			
Venlafaxine	37.5	75–225	300
Duloxetine	30	60–120	120
TCAs			
Clomipramine	25	100–150	250
Imipramine	25	100–150	300

Table 1.
Dosage of antidepressants effective in panic disorder.

5.2.1.2 Efficacy of antidepressants in long-term treatment of panic disorder

The SSRIs i.e., citalopram, fluvoxamine, paroxetine, the SNRIs venlafaxine and duloxetine and the TCAs, all remain effective in the treatment of panic disorder over the long-term [5, 15, 22, 52].

5.2.1.3 Side effects of antidepressants

In order to avoid or at least alleviate adverse effects, it is recommended that the starting daily dose of antidepressant drugs be lower than the recommended effective dose, and that the daily dose increase will be gradual in the first weeks of treatment. Psycho-education of patients with panic disorder about side effects and slow onset of action of antidepressants is very important. The assessment of outcome should be made only after several weeks of treatment.

5.2.1.4 Dropout rates in treatment of panic disorder with antidepressants

During pharmacological treatment of panic disorder 18% of patients treated with SSRIs, 1–12% of patients treated with venlafaxine and about 30% of patients treated with TCAs dropout prematurely [5, 50, 64].

5.2.2 Benzodiazepines

There are a number of clinical studies, with many years of experience, which indicated that benzodiazepines are effective in treating patients with panic disorders. The benzodiazepines are superior to placebo in the acute phase treatment of panic disorder [11, 63]. They have strong effects on somatic symptoms of anxiety and sleep problems. In addition, Benzodiazepines have a fast onset of action, i.e., they produce effects as soon as an effective dose is administered. For half an hour to an hour after taking benzodiazepine, panic symptoms are reduced, and patients feel easier. No other drug can do this [11]. The correct dosage of benzodiazepine involves a gradual increase in dose to a dose that removes symptoms and does not cause significant adverse effects, with regular taking more than once a day. Dosage of benzodiazepines effective in panic disorder is shown in **Table 2**.

5.2.2.1 Length of treatment with benzodiazepines

Due to the possible occurrence of dependence and abstinence syndrome, the duration of therapy with benzodiazepines should be short, for several weeks. However, because of the chronic character of the disease, sometimes they should be administered for several months, even for a year with continuous monitoring of the patient [47].

5.2.2.2 Side effects and risks involved in treatment with benzodiazepines

When benzodiazepines are prescribed for long-term use, dependence may occur manifested by dose escalation and problems withdrawing the medication [47, 63].

5.2.2.3 Dropout rates in treatment with benzodiazepines

In panic disorder trials, dropout rates due to side effects are about 15% for benzodiazepines [47].

5.2.3 First-line pharmacotherapy of panic disorder

SSRIs and venlafaxine should both be considered first-line agents for treatment of panic disorder. SSRIs and venlafaxine are effective in acute and long-term treatment, have an acceptable side effect profile and acceptable dropout rate [16, 48, 57].

TCAs may have a slower onset than SSRIs. In addition, TCAs have a less tolerable side effect profile than SSRIs given that they have more anticholinergic effects, and are generally less safe than SSRIs. Finally, reported dropout rates are higher for TCAs compared to SSRIs [5, 6, 62].

In summary, benzodiazepines as monotherapy should not be regarded as a first-line treatment in view of their side effect profile and in view of their lack of efficacy in treating comorbid conditions.

5.2.4 Optimal duration of pharmacotherapy of panic disorder

Studies reported that more than half of the patients interrupt treatment within several months to years [62, 64]. But considering, often relapsing course of panic disorder long-term treatment is recommended [3, 7, 12, 22, 43]. Most guidelines refer to expert consensus and suggest pharmacotherapy for at least a year [6].

Benzodiazepines			
Drug name	**Start**	**Recommended**	**Maximum**
Alprazolam	1	2–4	6
Clonazepam	0.25–0.5	1.5–3	6
Diazepam	5–10	40–50	50
Lorazepam	1–3	2.5–7.5	10
Bromazepam	3	3–9	15

Table 2.
Dosage of benzodiazepines effective in panic disorder.

Providing psychotherapy to panic disorder patients is also beneficial in enhancing the long-term outcome. Some evidence indicates that a CBT relapse-prevention program prevents relapse in patients with panic disorder [23, 59].

5.2.5 Pharmacotherapy in treatment-refractory patients with panic disorder

Some panic disorder patients do not respond, or only respond partially to pharmacotherapy. The treatment of refractory patients should consist of optimizing the current treatment, switching to another agent, or augmentation. Optimizing the current pharmacotherapy may be useful but some studies reported that an increased dosage of a SSRI is no more effective [8, 43].

Switching within or between classes of pharmacological agents, or to another treatment modality with proven efficacy in treating panic disorder, such as CBT, may be effective [23, 29, 53, 57].

Augmentation of antidepressants with an antipsychotic has been suggested for refractory panic disorder patients [30, 54, 56].

6. Conclusion

Panic disorder is a prevalent and disabling disorder with unknown etiology. Panic disorder should be diagnosed as soon as possible and to start the treatment which can be effective. The main treatment for panic disorder is psychotherapy and medication. One or both types of treatment may be recommended, depending of the patient preference, his history and the severity of the panic. The first-line treatment of panic disorder usually is CBT and pharmacotherapy with SSRIs. The recommendations are at least a year of antidepressant treatment. Management of treatment-refractory panic disorder includes a range of switching and augmentation strategies. Psychotherapy helps patients to overcome their fears usually within several months, but occasional visits afterward can help them to ensure that panic attacks are under control.

Conflict of interest

The authors declare that there is no conflict of interest.

Author details

Dimitar Bonevski and Andromahi Naumovska*
Faculty of Medicine, St. Cyril and Methodius, Skopje, North Macedonia

*Address all correspondence to: andromahi_n@yahoo.com

References

[1] Addis ME et al. Effectiveness of cognitive behavioral therapy for panic disorder versus treatment as usual in a managed care setting: 2-year follow-up. Journal of Consulting and Clinical Psychology. 2006;**74**:377-385

[2] Alaor SF. Does the association between mitral valve prolapse and panic disorder really exist? The Primary Care Companion to The Journal of Clinical Psychiatry. 2008;**10**(1):38-47

[3] APA. Practice Guidelines for the Treatment of Patients with Panic Disorder. 2nd ed. Washington, DC: American Psychiatric Association; 2009

[4] Baillie AJ, Rapee RM. Predicting who benefits from psychoeducation and self-help for panic attacks. Behaviour Research and Therapy. 2004;**42**:513-527

[5] Bakker A et al. SSRIs vs. TCAs in the treatment of panic disorder: A meta-analysis. Acta Psychiatrica Scandinavica. 2002;**106**:163-167

[6] Bandelow B et al. Meta-analysis of randomized controlled comparisons of psychopharmacological and psychological treatments for anxiety disorders. The World Journal of Biological Psychiatry. 2007;**8**:175-187

[7] Batelaan NM et al. The 2-year prognosis of panic episodes in the general population. Psychological Medicine. 2010;**40**:147-157

[8] Batelaan NM et al. Evidence-based pharmacotherapy of panic disorder: An update. The International Journal of Neuropsychopharmacology. 2012;**15**:403-415

[9] Bonevski D, Naumovska A. Trauma and anxiety disorders throughout lifespan: Fear and anxiety from normality to disorder. Psychiatria Danubina. 2018;**30**(Suppl 6):384-389

[10] Bonevski D. Child abuse in panic disorder. Medicinski Pregled. 2008;**61**(3-4):169-172

[11] Bruce SE et al. Are benzodiazepines still the medication of choice for patients with panic disorder with or without agoraphobia? American Journal of Psychiatry. 2003;**160**:1432-1438

[12] Choy Y et al. Three-year medication prophylaxis in panic disorder: To continue or discontinue? A naturalistic study. Comprehensive Psychiatry. 2007;**48**:419-425

[13] Cosci F et al. Cigarette smoking and panic: A critical review of the literature. The Journal of Clinical Psychiatry. 2010;**71**:606-615

[14] Craske MG, Barlow DH. Mastery of your Anxiety and Panic (Workbook). 4th ed. New York: Oxford University Press; 2007

[15] Crippa JA, Zuardi AW. Duloxetine in the treatment of panic disorder. International Journal of Neuropsychopharmacology. 2006;**9**:633-634

[16] Dannon PN et al. A naturalistic long-term comparison study of selective serotonin reuptake inhibitors in the treatment of panic disorder. Clinical Neuropharmacology. 2007;**30**:326-334

[17] Davidoff J et al. Quality of life in panic disorder: Looking beyond symptom remission. Quality of Life Research: An International Journal of Quality of Life Aspects of Treatment, Care and Rehabilitation. 2012;**21**:945-959

[18] De Jonge P et al. Cross-national epidemiology of panic disorder and panic attacks in the world mental health surveys. Depression and Anxiety. 2016;**33**(12):1155-1177

[19] Donovan MR et al. Comparative efficacy of antidepressants in preventing relapse in anxiety disorders—A meta-analysis. Journal of Affective Disorders. 2010;**123**:9-16

[20] Dresler T et al. Revise the revised? New dimensions of the neuroanatomical hypothesis of panic disorder. Journal of Neural Transmission (Vienna). 2013;**120**:3-29. DOI: 10.1007/s00702-012-0811-1

[21] Moitra E et al. Impact of stressful life events on the course of panic disorder in adults. Journal of Affective Disorders. 2011;**134**(1-3):373-376

[22] Ferguson JM et al. Relapse prevention of panic disorder in adult outpatient responders to treatment with venlafaxine extended release. The Journal of Clinical Psychiatry. 2007;**68**:58-68

[23] Furukawa TA, Watanabe N, Churchill R. Psychotherapy plus antidepressant for panic disorder with or without agoraphobia: Systematic review. British Journal of Psychiatry. 2006;**188**:305-312

[24] Goddard AW et al. Reductions in occipital cortex GABA levels in panic disorder detected with 1h-magnetic resonance spectroscopy. Archives of General Psychiatry. 2001;**58**:556-561

[25] Goodwin RD, Fergusson DM, Horwood LJ. Childhood abuse and familial violence and the risk of panic attacks and panic disorder in young adulthood. Psychological Medicine. 2005;**35**:881-890

[26] Ham BJ et al. Decreased GABA levels in anterior cingulate and basal ganglia in medicated subjects with panic disorder: A proton magnetic resonance spectroscopy (1H-MRS) study. Progress in Neuro-Psychopharmacology & Biological Psychiatry. 2007;**31**(2):403-411

[27] Harvison KW, Woodruff-Borden J, Jeffery SE. Mismanagement of panic disorder in emergency departments: Contributors, costs, and implications for integrated models of care. Journal of Clinical Psychology and Medicine. 2004;**11**:217-232

[28] Hasler G et al. Asthma and panic in young adults: A 20-year prospective community study. American Journal of Respiratory and Critical Care Medicine. 2005;**171**:1224-1230

[29] Heldt E et al. One-year follow-up of pharmacotherapy-resistant patients with panic disorder treated with cognitive-behavior therapy: Outcome and predictors of remission. Behavior Research and Therapy. 2006;**44**(5):657-665. DOI: 10.1016/j. brat.2005.05.003

[30] Hoge EA et al. Aripiprazole as augmentation treatment of refractory generalized anxiety disorder and panic disorder. CNS Spectrums. 2008;**13**:522-527

[31] Kalk NJ, Nutt DJ, Lingford-Hughes AR. The role of central noradrenergic dysregulation in anxiety disorders: Evidence from clinical studies. Journal of Psychopharmacology. 2008;**25**(1):3-16

[32] Kessler RC et al. The epidemiology of panic attacks, panic disorder, and agoraphobia in the National Comorbidity Survey Replication. Archives of General Psychiatry. 2006;**63**:415-424

[33] Kessler RC et al. The epidemiology of panic attacks, panic disorder, and agoraphobia in the national comorbidity survery replication. Archives of General Psychiatry. 2006;**63**:415-424

[34] Kikuchi M. Relationship between anxiety and thyroid function in patients with panic disorder. Progress in Neuro-Psychopharmacology & Biological Psychiatry. 2005;**29**(1):77-81

[35] Kjernisted K, McIntosh D. Venlafaxine extended release (XR) in the treatment of panic disorder. Therapeutics and Clinical Risk Management. 2007;**3**:59-69

[36] Kuijpers PM et al. Panic disorder in patients with chest pain and palpitations: An often unrecognized relationship. Nederlands Tijdschrift voor Geneeskunde. 2000;**144**:732-736

[37] Latas M et al. Farmakoterapija u Psihijatrii. Beograd: Cedup; 2018

[38] Liebowitz MR, Asnis G, Mangano R, Tzanis E. A double-blind, placebo-controlled, parallel-group, flexible-dose study of venlafaxine extended release capsules in adult outpatients with panic disorder. Journal of Clinical Psychiatry. 2009;**70**(4):550-561

[39] Lotufo-Neto F et al. A dose-finding and discontinuation study of clomipramine in panic disorder. Journal of Psychopharmacology. 2001;**15**:13-17

[40] Maron E, Hettema JM, Shlik J. Advances in molecular genetics of panic disorder. Molecular Psychiatry. 2010;**15**:681-701

[41] Maron E, Shlik J. Serotonin function in panic disorder: Important, but why? Neuropsychopharmacology. 2006;**31**(1):1-11

[42] Martin EI et al. The neurobiology of anxiety disorders: Brain imaging, genetics, and psychoneuroendocrinology. The Psychiatric Clinics of North America. 2009;**32**:549-575

[43] McIntyre JS et al. Practice Guideline for the Treatment of Patients with Panic Disorder. 2nd ed. Arlington, VA: American Psychiatric Association; 2009

[44] Meuret AE et al. Do unexpected panic attacks occur spontaneously? Biological Psychiatry. 2011;**70**:985-991. DOI: 10.1016/j.biopsych.2011.05.027

[45] Milrod BL et al. Manual of Panic-Focused Psychodynamic Psychotherapy. Washington, DC: American Psychiatric Press; 1997

[46] Muideen A. Pharmacologic Management of Acute and Chronic Panic Disorder. US Pharmacist. 2015;**40**(11):HS24-HS30

[47] Offidani E et al. Efficacy and tolerability of benzodiazepines versus antidepressants in anxiety disorders: A systematic review and meta-analysis. Psychotherapy and Psychosomatics. 2013;**82**:355-362

[48] Otto MW et al. An effect-size analysis of the relative efficacy and tolerability of serotonin selective reuptake inhibitors for panic disorder. The American Journal of Psychiatry. 2001;**158**:1989-1992

[49] Otto MW, Deveney C. Cognitive-behavioral therapy and the treatment of panic disorder: Efficacy and strategies. Journal of Clinical Psychiatry. 2005;**66**:28-32

[50] Perna G et al. Long-term pharmacological treatments of anxiety disorders: An updated systematic review. Current Psychiatry Reports. 2016;**18**:23

[51] Porter E, Chambless DL. A systematic review of predictors and moderators of improvement in cognitive-behavioral therapy for panic disorder and agoraphobia. Clinical Psychology Review. 2015;**42**:179-192. DOI: 10.1016/j.cpr.2015.09.004

[52] Rapaport MH et al. Sertraline treatment of panic disorder: Results of a long-term study. Acta Psychiatrica Scandinavica. 2001;**104**:289-298

[53] Rodrigues H et al. CBT for pharmacotherapy non-remitters—A systematic review of a next-step strategy. Journal of Affective Disorders. 2011;**129**:219-228

[54] Saito M, Miyaoka H. Augmentation of paroxetine with clocapramine in panic disorder. Psychiatry and Clinical Neurosciences. 2007;**61**:449

[55] Schumacher J et al. The genetics of panic disorder. Journal of Medical Genetics. 2011;**48**:361-368

[56] Sepede G et al. Olanzapine augmentation in treatment-resistant panic disorder: A 12-week, fixed-dose, open-label trial. Journal of Clinical Psychopharmacology. 2006;**26**(1):45-49

[57] Simon NM et al. Next-step strategies for panic disorder refractory to initial pharmacotherapy: A 3-phase randomized clinical trial. The Journal of Clinical Psychiatry. 2009;**70**(11):1563-1570

[58] Simon NM et al. Open-label support for duloxetine for the treatment of panic disorder. CNS Neuroscience & Therapeutics. 2009;**15**(1):19-23. DOI: 10.1111/j.1755-5949.2008.00076.x

[59] Smits JAJ, O'Cleirigh CM, Otto MW. Combining cognitive-behavioral therapy and pharmacotherapy for the treatment of panic disorder. Journal of Cognitive Psychotherapy. 2006;**20**:75-84

[60] Spatola C et al. Gene–environment interactions in panic disorder and CO_2 sensitivity: Effects of events occurring early in life. American Journal of Medical Genetics. Part B, Neuropsychiatric Genetics. 2011;**79-88**(34):56

[61] Stahl SM, Gergel I, Li D. Escitalopram in the treatment of panic disorder: A randomized, double-blind, placebo-controlled trial. Journal of Clinical Psychiatry. 2003;**64**:1322-1327

[62] Stein MB et al. Antidepressant adherence and medical resource use among managed care patients with anxiety disorders. Psychiatric Services. 2006;**57**:673-680

[63] Susman J, Klee B. The role of high-potency benzodiazepines in the treatment of panic disorder prim care companion. The Journal of Clinical Psychiatry. 2005;**7**(1):5-11

[64] Toni C et al. Spontaneous treatment discontinuation in panic disorder patients treated with antidepressants. Acta Psychiatrica Scandinavica. 2004;**110**:130-137

[65] Van Rijn B, Wild C. Humanistic and integrative therapies for anxiety and depression: Practice-based evaluation of transactional analysis, gestalt and integrative psychotherapies and person centered counseling. Transactional Analysis Journal. 2013;**43**(2):150-163. DOI: 10.1177/036253713499545

[66] Weissman M. Family genetic studies of panic disorder. Journal of Psychiatric Research. 1993;**27**(1):69-78

[67] Wesner C et al. Effect of cognitive-behavioral group therapy for panic disorder in changing coping strategies. Comprehensive Psychiatry. 2013;**55**(1):87-92. DOI: 10.1016/j.comppsych.2013.06.008

Chapter 9

Anxiety: The Dizziness of Freedom—The Developmental Factors of Anxiety as Seen through the Lens of Psychoanalytic Thinking

Peter Slater

Abstract

This chapter explores how anxiety is necessary for development to take place. It explores the link between Soren Kierkegaard's existential views on anxiety with more recent psychoanalytic theories on anxiety as espoused by Sigmund Freud, Melanie Klein and Wilfred Bion in particular. The chapter postulates that an optimal degree of anxiety is more likely to be obtained by access, in early life, to a mind (often a parental figure) that is able to offer a containing and transformative function to the infant's primitive destructive impulses and resultant fears and anxieties. Clinical examples are included to demonstrate the role of psychotherapy in providing an alternative containing presence that can tolerate and transform severe states of anxiety.

Keywords: anxiety, containment, projective identification, persecutory anxiety, depressive anxiety, development

1. Introduction

In 1844, Soren Kierkegaard [1] wrote of anxiety as being the 'dizziness of freedom', the dizzying effect of looking into the boundlessness of one's own possibilities. Without anxiety there would be no possibility and therefore no capacity to grow and develop as a human being.

This chapter will examine psychoanalytic concepts of anxiety, in particular those of Sigmund Freud and key figures in the British School of Object Relations Melanie Klein and Wilfred Bion. It will demonstrate the close links between psychoanalytic theories on anxiety and the existential thinking about anxiety as espoused by Kierkegaard. The chapter will look at how the role and function of anxiety is an important determinant in the development of symbolic functioning, in creativity and most crucially in the origins of thought and thinking.

Clinical vignettes and material taken from psychoanalytic psychotherapy with children and teenagers will be drawn upon in order to extrapolate thinking about anxiety that is in the service of growth and development (possibility) and the unbounded anxiety which undermines and can arrest personality development, potentially leading to psychopathology.

IntechOpen

2. Kierkegaard and anxiety as the dizziness of freedom

Mawson [2] contends that 'Anxiety informs us of our being, anxiety being stimulated by contact with primordial truths. It is in relation to anxiety that we are helped by other human beings to bear what is and what we are'. Central to this exploration of anxiety is the idea that if we are able to endure and to stay with painful emotional experience, then we are likely to be able to grow from it. Fundamentally, this process of staying with the difficult charts an ontological journey from a state of 'knowing to being'. On this point, Mawson refers to Bion's [3] memories of homesickness when he was sent away to boarding school in another country as a young boy. Bion described the experience as being akin to a 'horrible impending disaster' with no words to adequately describe it:

One might write an anthology but it would require skill, almost amounting to genius, to begin to recall the absolute dread that comes on those occasions. But I believe it is from one's ability to stand having such feelings and ideas that mental growth eventually comes.

For the purposes of this chapter, our exploration of anxiety begins with Soren Kierkegaard's own interest in the part played by anxiety in the emotional life of the individual. Kierkegaard [1] placed anxiety alongside dread and angst, viewing it as unfocused fear. In his thinking about anxiety, he wrote of a man standing on the edge of a cliff, who when looking over the edge experiences a visceral fear of falling, but what accompanies this fear is also a terrifying impulse to intentionally throw himself off the edge. Kierkegaard posited that this is an experience of anxiety or dread because it puts us in touch with the very nature of possibility, in other words to choose to do one thing or another—in this case to stay firmly rooted to the ledge or to throw oneself off it. What was striking to Kierkegaard was the individual's complete freedom to choose one's options; it is this freedom to choose (even if it is the most terrifying of all options open to us) that creates dread and anxiety. Kierkegaard thus formulated anxiety as being the 'dizziness of freedom'.

In Kierkegaard's thinking, anxiety informs us of the choices we have at hand. He takes as his starting point the biblical example of Adam who was faced with the choice as whether to eat from the forbidden tree of knowledge in the Garden of Eden or to refrain. Adam was not aware of good or evil, right or wrong, but Kierkegaard emphasises that anxiety is born when Adam, knowing of God's prohibition about eating from the tree, still chooses to eat from it. Kierkegaard recognised the damning nature for mankind of Adam eating from the tree but also asserted the positive value of the idea that anxiety informs humankind of the choices we have at hand. This infers growth in the form of an opportunity to become self-aware, the need for personal responsibility and the potential for learning and growing from experience. What is pivotal to the more contemporary study of anxiety is how Kierkegaard viewed anxiety, as an opportunity for growth from a more self-centred need for immediacy to a more self-reflective, self-conscious state. Kierkegaard [1] wrote:

'Whoever has learned to be anxious in the right way, has learned the ultimate... Anxiety is freedom's possibility, and only such anxiety is through faith absolutely educative, because it consumes all finite ends and discovers all their deceptiveness. And no Grand Inquisitor such dreadful torments in readiness as anxiety has, and no secret agent knows as cunningly as anxiety to attack his suspect in his weakest moment or to make alluring the trap in which he will be caught, and no discerning judge understands how to interrogate and examine the accused as does anxiety, which never lets the accused escape, neither through amusement, nor by noise, not during work, neither by day or night'.

It is the idea that through anxiety not only can the individual become truly aware of their potential but that anxiety can also lead to an awareness of one's own true identity and sense of freedom. Kierkegaard's philosophy of anxiety is a useful point of origin to the later thinking of Sigmund Freud, and more contemporary psychoanalysts, on the subject of anxiety. The subject of anxiety has occupied a central place in psychoanalytic thinking and practice from its inception. Mawson [2] goes as far as to suggest that the principle premise is that from the beginning of life, it is in relation to anxiety that we are helped to bear the painful nature of reality and truth.

2.1 Psychoanalytic perspectives on anxiety

Freud placed anxiety at the centre of psychic[1] functioning and in so doing described anxiety as the greatest burden we face as a species. His proclamation was that because of the inexorable conflict between the life and death instincts, feelings of anxiety were inevitable. Freud's inherent belief was that development and growth can only occur with a degree of psychic pain and anxiety. His early theories centred upon the various means by which the mind defended itself against unbearable levels of anxiety, which if left unchecked became a state or experience of profound 'unpleasure'. He initially believed that anxiety was due to the build-up of internal tension, of instinctual impulses (often sexual in nature), that were unable to be released (expressed), often transforming into psychosomatic disturbances. Freud's view was that the inherent motivation of the individual is towards the discharge of such instinctual tensions. We can see this in the example of a 16-year-old female, who I will call Jess. Jess came for ongoing psychoanalytic psychotherapy due to severe self-harming behaviours and suicidal ideation. During the early part of our work, she spoke of the unbearable emotional pain that built up and threatened to overwhelm her. She described the pain coming from inside, building up into a crescendo, whose only relief was through cutting and self-harm. She once explained that physical pain was much more bearable than the inside, emotional pain, which appeared to lessen when she could feel pain in her body.

Jess's material captures the essence of the need not only to defend against overwhelming internal states of anxiety, dread and despair but also the strong desire to discharge this tension by any means possible. Freud posited that the human nervous system had a strong propensity to flee from anything painful. An important function of psychotherapy can be thought of as providing a therapeutic space for the patient to begin to put unthinkable thoughts into words and to begin to bear or tolerate unbearable emotional states. It is this process that can offer an alternative to the 'acting out' of such feelings in repetitive or compulsive ways and an alternative to a propensity to flee or discharge emotions in self-destructive or depriving ways as with Jess above. Anxiety is, as Kierkegaard reminds us, the awareness of a freedom to choose, which in itself can lead to a growth in self-awareness and self-reflection. This is only possible if anxiety can be borne by both the patient and the therapist and by both mother-figure and infant.

In 1926, Freud [4] put his second theory of anxiety forwards. In this theory he described how anxiety acts as a danger sign to the ego[2] alerting it to the impending

[1] Psychoanalytic theory uses the word psychic to describe a dynamic internal state or reality, which can be at odds with external reality. Psychic or psychical is therefore pertaining to the internal world of the individual.

[2] In psychoanalytic terms the ego is defined as the part of the self that deals with external reality and is central to the process of integration of the personality as a whole. In the infant the ego is understandably weak and rudimentary in its formation and development and therefore at the mercy of anxiety and internal tension, experienced as something painfully physical or bodily.

endangerment of a traumatic or perilous situation. In this theory Freud emphasises the danger situation as coming from a separation or loss of a loved object. This was to become the basis of Melanie Klein's later thinking on primitive anxiety states in the infant. What is prominent in much of Freud's early thinking on anxiety is the relationship between external and internal sources of anxiety, consonant with both is the survival of the organism, either physically or psychically (internal, emotional survival). The idea is being that the separation or loss of the loved object could be a concrete, external experience which galvanises anxiety or an internal experience, a feeling or thought about loss that is equally anxiety-provoking.

Freud [5] described the infant's experiences of hunger or a feeling of dying as potentially leading to severe states of suffering and anxiety. We might wonder whether Freud was linking this infantile state of hunger and fear of dying with the experience of abandonment, separation or loss of something life-giving. Freud recognised that the infant's efforts to dispel and evacuate such overwhelming fears and anxieties about its very survival (often in the form of cries, screams, bodily evacuations, muscular tensing) were not always possible for the infant to achieve by itself. As touched upon above, the infant very much depends on help from another in managing such anxiety states and help usually provided by the mother or mother-figure. Indeed, Freud saw the basic human unit as that of the mother-infant couple. He posited that it is the mother-figure as an outside helper that provides timely and appropriate intervention to help the infant manage internal states and tensions, which generate overwhelming levels of fear and anxiety for the infant's immature ego to manage alone.

Freud's initial idea of placing anxiety at the centre of the development of the self, along with the concomitant array of defences that the mind mobilises to ameliorate anxiety, was taken further by post-Freudian thinkers, no more so than by Meanie Klein. Klein made more explicitly the role and function of anxiety both in the service of growth and development and also in terms of pathology and mental illness.

2.2 Klein's two forms of anxiety

Freud's theory of the unconscious realm of the mind was arguably his greatest legacy. He postulated that much of our emotional experience, much of our behaviour, did not originate in our conscious or rational mind, but was instead formed in a deeply dynamic, unconscious domain. Freud pointed to dreams; to slips of the tongue; to the transference (attributing to the therapist qualities that belong often to a parent or an internal state of mind, thought or feeling); and to projective mechanisms that particularly occur between patient and psychotherapist as evidence of such an unconscious realm. It is where the perpetual tussle takes place between instincts in the service of life and survival and those inexorably pulling towards stagnation and death.

Such theoretical underpinnings were taken and developed by Melanie Klein, whose work in the 1920s–1940s with children as young as 3 years old led her to conclude, in line with Freud, that anxiety originates from an internal fear of annihilation, fragmentation and falling apart. Klein [6] wrote:

There is in the unconscious a fear of annihilation of life. Thus in my view the danger arising from the inner working of the death instinct is the first cause of anxiety. This source of anxiety is never eliminated and enters as a perpetual factor into all anxiety situations.

In her clinical work as a psychoanalyst working with children, Klein placed the interpretation and understanding of anxiety states in the child at the epicentre of her psychoanalytic method. Klein's work with children illustrated how powerful a child's anxieties were, anxieties that were often at the core of their difficulties in feeding, sleeping and learning. By interpreting the child's strongest anxieties and fears in the consulting room (while referring back to the earliest objects that populate the child's internal world), Klein found that anxiety could be alleviated. She also observed from her analytic work with children how development that had been heavily impinged upon by such anxieties could gradually become unstuck leading to a more age-appropriate developmental trajectory. Creative mental processes, such as symbol formation and personification, which allow for an 'as if' quality to our psychological world, can be best viewed in a child's play. These are observed as the child undertakes a process of attributing internal states of mind, feeling and cognitive states, to toy figures and animals and to play scenarios, which the lessening of anxiety can set in motion.

Sarah[3], a 4-year-old, was referred by her parents for psychoanalytic child psychotherapy due to their concerns about her preoccupation with eating, an inability to separate from her mother and to engage socially with others in an age-appropriate way. The mother spoke of her own considerable battle, following Sarah's birth, with postnatal depression, which she described as at times being quite debilitating.

Sarah's fixation with food was quite overwhelming for her parents, whose trips out as a family were dominated by Sarah's need to know when and where they would eat on their trip. Her day, and thereby the family's day, was organised around when the next meal time would be. She demonstrated a good deal of omnipotent behaviour, dominating and bossing her parents and breaking down into floods of tears if she did not have her needs immediately met. The mother described how she could not do anything at home without Sarah needing to be with her. Sarah found it impossible to play alone with her toys, for example, and dropping Sarah off at the nursery was described as a 'nightmare' situation by both parents. A typical scene was of Sarah clinging to her mother's legs, begging her not to leave her; when she did try to leave, she often ended up dragging Sarah along the floor with her as she tried to get to the door. Sarah's mother did wonder if her own struggles with depression had had an impact on her daughter.

In the consulting room with Sarah, these situations were enacted in her play and her need to have me ever-present in the play with her was striking. After five sessions, Sarah had been able to come into the room on her own, but only if her mother was standing outside the door. Sarah would say she needed the toilet in order to gain access to her mother, so great was the anxiety of separating from her. In this early part of our work, Sarah would implore me to play with her, falling down in a heap when I informed her that I needed to think about what she was doing in the room. She would even announce on the way to the consulting room the order of things we were to do in our session that day, activities that would inevitably involve both of us. The play often centred on food, feeding and making food with playdough and a repeated scene of going to a café. Even in her play, Sarah found it hard to share, and I would need to be the one deprived and left without. Her food was greedily and ravenously eaten, something parents had said was evident wherever Sarah ate her food.

In this example, the intolerable aspects of a young child's anxiety about separation heavily flavour much of the clinical material. The overwhelming need not to leave any gaps or spaces when eating or when playing was palpable. If there was any gap or a lull, the terrifying fear was of her psychically, internally, falling down it with nothing there to break her fall. It was evident how such levels of anxiety,

---

[3] Names and any identifying details of patients in all of these vignettes have all been anonymised for purposes of maintaining confidentiality.

seemingly generated from within and part of her internal unconscious world, have markedly impinged upon her age-appropriate functioning. This was particularly evident in her capacity to play on her own and to share with others. Wanting sole possession of her mother and the anxiety generated by her potential absence was a primary feature, filling the gaps meant avoiding separation. We might think of the preoccupation with food and the need to eat continually as a defence against the painful separation from mummy's feeding presence (the breast/bottle). Indeed, Sarah's behaviours generally appeared in the service of defending against the unbearable anxiety evoked by separation. The omnipotent, demanding, bossy behaviour ensured close proximity to her object, yet such defences had a huge impact on her emotional and social development.

What is crucial to an understanding of this process is Klein's formulation of two different forms of anxiety (persecutory and depressive anxieties), which have as their point of origin the first loved object[4] or object relationship with that of the mother's breast[5]. Klein elaborated upon Freud's idea of the unconscious realm to view all mental life of the individual as originating from the unconscious. Sexual, aggressive, loving, hating impulses all go to make up the internal world of unconscious phantasy, colouring and flavouring how we see and relate to the world out there as well as the world inside.

Mawson [2] points to Joan Riviere's [7] work on unconscious phantasy to bring descriptive meaning to such a visceral part of the mind:

The inner world is exclusively one of personal relations, in which nothing is external, in the sense that everything happening in it refers to the self, to the individual in whom it is part. It is formed solely on the basis of the individual's own desires towards other persons and of his reactions to them as objects of his desires.

2.3 Persecutory anxiety

According to Klein, the infant's early relationship to the mother is of a part-object nature; the breast or feeding part is seen as the infant's own possession. The breast[6] can only be related to a binary form—it is a good object when it is present and offering a fulfilling feed or frustrating and bad when it is absent and the phantasy is of it feeding another. We can see how this picture captures the quality of how Sarah is related to her object, for example, in the last session before a holiday break, Sarah took me by the hand and led me to the corner of the room. She said sharply that I was now in gaol and would need to stay there until she comes back from the holiday. Again, it is crucial to understand this primitive form of relating to the object as part of the infant's unconscious phantasy[7], experienced in primitive terms of bodily pleasure, fulfilment, being filled up or conversely in terms of hunger, pain, emptiness and annihilation when the breast or mother is absent. For Sarah

[4] In psychoanalytic terms 'an object' can be an internal entity based loosely on experiences of and with external parental/familial figures. Early experiences with parental figures are taken inside (introjected), installed and identified with internally. An internal object is not an exact replica of the external parent-figure as the infant's own unique constitutional makeup will flavour the quality of the object and the way the object is taken in.

[5] I am using the term mother to describe one of the primary figures in this mother-infant relationship, but it could also be a mother-figure in the shape of a father, partner, grandparent, etc.

[6] The breast or the bottle is interchangeable here, and the intention is not to promote breast-feeding as superior to bottle feeding. Breast is therefore interchangeable in this chapter with bottle.

[7] Phantasy with 'ph' in psychoanalytic thinking denotes an unconscious process and idea, whereas fantasy denotes a thought, idea and day-dream that we are more conscious of.

putting me in gaol was a way of keeping me (the breast) away from other children whom I might see in her absence, she could lock me, having exclusive access to me when she needs a therapeutic feed as it were.

From the work with young children, whose anxieties were such a strong feature of their challenging presentations, Klein developed the concept of projective identification. This is a seminal concept that underpins much of the work and understanding of unconscious aspects of relationships in psychoanalytic theory and practice. It is a concept that links back to Freud's idea of the infant who expels unbearable pain, anxiety or fear. Klein believed that it was the breast or the mother-figure who would be the recipient or receptacle for these unwanted experiences of the infant. The cries, screams and bodily expulsions are the means by which the infant projects into the object, but for Klein the process of evacuation of such unpleasurable sensations does not conclude this process. The projection of unwanted states, thoughts, feelings and experiences is not solely consigned to the infant; it is a defensive process that we all adopt at times of high anxiety in particular. Klein, however, observed that an object that is projected into is changed and can be affected by the content of what is projected into it. For the infant, the primitive experience of such a projection into the breast of its frustration, hatred, anger and aggression (because of its absence) is that the breast or object now becomes identified with such feelings. It takes the form of an angry, aggressive, vengeful breast, thus turning suddenly into a terrifying entity that is hell-bent on revenge. We could argue that for Sarah when the breast or feeding mother or adult figure was present, it was a benign, safe, fulfilling object, but when absent it was not just a withholding object but a terrifyingly bad and insidious object that wanted to starve her to death. The anxiety this generated in Sarah was to such a degree that certain areas of her psychosocial and emotional development were arrested.

This anxiety Klein [5] termed is 'persecutory anxiety'. It has a strong paranoid flavour, defences in what she called 'paranoid-schizoid phase' of development, including the splitting of the object (breast) into good and bad, the omnipotent projection into the object of unwanted emotional and physical sensations and a fervent denial of reality. This phase is one of the self-concerns of the undifferentiated states with the mother or mother-figure perceived only as an extension of the infant's self. Persecutory anxiety is therefore of a very primitive nature, archaic in that it reaches back to a time of an unintegrated internal state, the self or ego is disparate, easily fragmented and as Freud perceived, needing the help of another to hold it together when it is present. When it is not present, anxieties are heightened, and as what we saw with Sarah, the good object now becomes a bad, hating the one that can destroy and annihilate the self.

Klein [8] sees the importance of anxiety in this phase as being the origins of curiosity[8] which broadens outwards from the self-orientated preoccupation with the first object (the mother and the insides of her body) to objects in the outside world. It is the very fear of the persecuting objects that we have attacked in phantasy that impel us to seek solace in objects further afield. These outside objects become symbols for the original objects they stand for, for example, the mother's breast and her insides. There is a growing interest in new objects, but Klein argued if anxiety is too great, there is no symbolic replacement of one with another. As with Sarah, the incessant need for food and her preoccupation with food in our sessions was not standing for the mother's breast but was in her mind the concrete equivalence of her mother's breast (feeding capacity). I suspected that what enabled her to be present in the consulting room, without her mother's actual presence, was some capacity to play at making food or eating food, thus keeping her mother present in her own

---

[8] Klein called this the epistemophilic instinct—the desire to know.

mind through the symbolic representation of her mother. What was evident was how precarious this capacity was and how easily symbolic functioning (her play) could break down when anxiety levels became intolerable. At these moments the substitute for the mother was not enough she needed the reassurance of the physical presence of her actual mother.

For Sarah, as with any 4-year-old, we would not expect her to be able to manage such severe anxieties by herself. However, we would think that in Sarah's case she was still stuck in Klein's paranoid-schizoid position and finding it very difficult to move forwards into the more developmentally mature phase or position which Klein [9] termed the depressive position.

2.4 Depressive anxiety

Halton [10], succinctly, describes Klein's idea of the depressive position and the central anxiety which emerges. He suggests that the anxiety here is as a result of a profound fear that the aggressiveness of the earlier paranoid-schizoid position has irreparably damaged the good object (mother-figure), leading in phantasy to the death of this life-giving source. This phase is flavoured, therefore, with feelings of guilt and remorse and a depressive form of anxiety which galvanises a need to repair the damage done to the object in phantasy. Halton suggests that the depressive position is characterised by a process of ego integration, of bringing different experiences together and of giving up the simplistic state of self-idealisation. It faces the growing self with the complex nature of internal and external reality, for example, that it is the same mother that fulfils that can also frustrate and withhold. The shift, we could say, is that from concern for the self to concern about the other.

Klein [11] emphasises the importance for the psychological well-being of the individual of reaching this developmental stage of the depressive position and how the anxiety of having damaged something precious stimulates a desire for work and creativity in the process of trying to repair. For Jess, a long and challenging therapeutic process exhibited a growing capacity to tolerate anxiety states. There was a growing ability to find more creative, symbolic ways of managing internal pain, namely, by giving words and language to it. With this articulation came a growing curiosity about how her mother battles with alcohol abuse, her father's early abandonment of the family and an ability to see the impact of past events on her present emotional experience. The need for self-harming behaviour diminished as she recognised she had more 'choices' to deal with the internal pain.

We see the importance Klein places on tolerating anxiety and the shift to 'depressive anxiety' in the development of the personality. In terms of the individual's capacity for thinking, for functioning symbolically and creatively, the ego has to develop a true relation to reality and to be able to '... tolerate the pressure of the earliest anxiety-situations. And as usual it is a question of a certain optimum balance of factors concerned. A sufficient quantity of anxiety is the necessary basis for an abundance of symbol formation and of phantasy: an adequate capacity of the ego to tolerate anxiety is essential if anxiety is to be satisfactorily worked over ... [8].

In both Jess and Sarah, we might argue that at the outset of the work, there was a limited capacity for tolerating anxiety. There was a greater need to 'act out', to evacuate and to get rid of the overwhelming levels of anxiety or to find sustenance and relief from the needed actual presence of the mother-figure. This acting out was often apparent in the therapeutic work, Jess at one point even harming herself in the clinic prior to her session with myself. Bearing my shock, my disappointment, my anger and my thinking about such feelings was an instrumental factor in the therapeutic process. Jess, at this stage of our work, could not tolerate and acquire for herself an 'optimum degree' of anxiety—the mind of another was still needed to provide this for her. This leads us onto the seminal work of Bion and his concept of container/contained. Bion recognised the importance of the openness of the mother's mind to understanding her child and the similar important quality of the psychotherapist's mind to the understanding of that of their patient's.

2.5 Wilfred Bion's concept of a container for the contained

It was the work of Bion that was instrumental in highlighting the need for another to manage anxiety, an idea initially conceptualised by Sigmund Freud. Mawson [2] comments on how Freud pointed towards not only the infant being unable to manage anxiety alone but that anxiety can be made bearable by '... .the timely intervention of the mother, orienting herself not only in the realm of the satisfaction of basic needs but, crucially in the domain of anxiety'. Mawson reminds us that the prototype for all anxiety is one based upon helplessness in the face of destructive forces from within, which the intervention by the mother is essential in helping to manage. It could be said that the infant's continued psychological existence depends heavily upon the mother's intervention in assuaging such primitive anxieties as those discussed above.

Bion [12] was able to recognise that the role of the mother surpassed the necessary provision of basic needs—feeding and physical comfort. Crucially, it also provided a containing function for the infant's anxiety. Bion took this initial idea further and saw that the containing experience of the mother might also be the kernel for the development of thought, thinking and learning. According to Mawson [2], Bion experienced this primary containing function of the mind as a 'dynamic living system'.

Through his clinical work with psychotic and schizophrenic patients in the 1940s–1950s, Bion developed further Klein's idea of projective identification[9] extending it beyond the need to get rid of unwanted emotional states or parts of the self. Projective identification in psychoanalytic terms is seen as an important process of maintaining an emotional equilibrium. It could be seen as a mechanism for releasing tension caused by anxiety that builds as a result of destructive feeling states from within. By placing these outside the self, attributing them elsewhere, the external object acts as a repository for them. Bion [12] felt that clinically projective identification by the patient could also be a useful tool for the psychotherapist in terms of it acting as a form of communication. Unthinkable, intolerable, emotional elements and parts of the self projected into the psychotherapist could be a useful tool to gain insight and an understanding of the patient's internal world. It could lend meaning to the patient's emotional experiences which were so intolerable and overwhelming that they needed to be expelled and forcefully put elsewhere.

Bion [13] describes the process of the mother accepting the infant's projective identifications, acting as a willing container that offers flexibility and a transformational process to the infant's anxieties around its own survival. It is the earliest form of communication as the mother receives the baby's distress, mulling it over in her mind to understand what the baby, through its distress and the impact on her, is letting her know. A simple example is the baby whose distress has made an impact on the mother, who in her containing function applies her own thinking as to why the baby might

[9] As discussed earlier, projective identification is an unconscious process, whereby unwanted emotions or parts of ourselves are split off, projected and now located in the other. The other is changed by this projection and is now seen as the embodiment of the anger, aggression, envy or other aspects that have been got rid of. It is the other that is angry, aggressive, frightening or envious, not our self. Good qualities/attributes can also be projected and left in others, often as a means of keeping such good aspects safe and away from destructive internal elements of the self.

be distressed. Working this out and meeting the babies need at that moment leads on a proto level to the baby feeling understood. To Bion's mind, it was the origin of the process of thinking and thought as provided by the thinking mind of another.

Bion [13] writes that the infant's projective identifications '... .arouse in the mother feelings which the infant wishes to be rid, if the infant feels it is dying it can arouse fears in the mother that it is dying. A well-balanced mother can accept these and respond therapeutically: that is to say in a manner that makes the infant feel it is receiving its frightened personality back again, but in a form that it can tolerate- the fears are manageable by the infant personality.

Bion is suggesting that it is the capacity of the mother, repeatedly, to bear the infant's unprocessed, unthinkable thoughts and intolerable feelings projected into her (the mother's processing of them and returning them back in a more tolerable form) that will eventually lead to the infant themselves taking in this containing capacity to think about and to reflect upon. Initially therefore, the mother is a 'thinker for the thoughts', until the infant develops the capacity (through repeated experiences of this process being provided by the mother) to think about the thoughts for themselves. This is the process of internalisation of an experience.

If the mother/mother-figure can tolerate the infant's projections and thereby provide such a containing function to the infants intolerable anxieties (without recourse to sending these projections back unprocessed and unmodified), then the infant will later become more able to tolerate, to stay with and to refine states of anxiety. Of course, Bion is saying much more than this. He refers more explicitly to the quality of this containing function of the parent as being essential for emotional, cognitive and psychosocial development. He also pointed to the dire consequences for development as a whole, if the parent is unwilling or unavailable to receive the infant's projections. This would therefore lead to an intolerance of difficult feelings and to increased levels of projection. Behaviour will be motivated by a greater need to expel, to avoid or to evade mental pain than to stay with and modify. Bion [13] turns to Keats when describing the role of the mother/therapist's capacity to tolerate the intolerable. Keats [14] described a concept of 'negative capability' ... that is, when a man is capable of being in uncertainties, mysteries, doubts, without any irritable reaching after fact and reason'.

We might wonder if Jess and Sarah had received a consistent enough experience of such a containing transformation of early anxieties. It should be kept in mind that these were parents who themselves struggled with their own very significant mental health difficulties, often in the absence of meaningful support from others. However, unlike their parents, both Jess and Sarah had come into contact with the containing presence and function of ongoing psychotherapy. Over time, Jess's self-harming ceased; she was better able to empathise with her mother's own difficult history as opposed to resorting to attacking and blaming her mother for her shortcomings. Jess found the potential within her to complete her studies and go onto university. Sarah did eventually find it easier to separate from her mother, to engage in creative and imaginative play and to share her play with her peers. The most pleasing for the parents was the broadening of her interests to include swimming and gymnastics, which signalled a shift away from her fixation with food and eating. This psychotherapeutic function corresponds with that of the mother-figure, of providing a mutative, containing function for the patient, a feeding back in a more processed form, through interpretation, those intolerable anxiety-ridden states. This process makes such states more bearable; it is a curative process that can lead to symbol formation, creativity and thinking. I can think about and put words to my worst fears and anxieties rather than acting them out in a ritualised or repetitive way.

Widening our focal point slightly, we might wish to turn to experimental psychology and in particular the seminal work of Yerkes and Dodson [11], Yerkes-Dodson law, to further illuminate Sarah and Jess's struggles with anxiety. As Kierkegaard [1] writes of the 'right kind of anxiety, the Yerkes-Dodson law suggests that there is a need for a 'right'-level of physiological and mental arousal (anxiety) for us to optimally perform certain tasks. The law suggests that challenging or cognitively demanding tasks may require lower levels of arousal in order to optimise concentration levels, whereas tasks that need physical stamina and perseverance may need higher levels of arousal. We might therefore wonder if the capacities of these two young people to develop both cognitively and emotionally were impacted upon by inappropriate levels of arousal given the areas of development under consideration. This is an interesting concept and one that as a psychotherapist it is worth considering in terms of the quality of therapeutic interventions. A therapeutic intervention might inadvertently serve to increase arousal levels in the patient when what is needed for the task is an intervention that offers the opposite. It is consistent with the idea that at times the patient needs the therapist to hear and understand (and not help the patient make sense of their experience) which may lower arousal levels and increase performance levels regarding focus and concentration, whereas there are other times that what is needed by the patient is for themselves to understand their internal/external experiences or states of mind with the help of the therapist which may be helped by an increase in arousal levels.

3. Conclusion

The emerging theme of this exploration of anxiety is that in order to allow ourselves the experience of Kierkegaard's [1] 'dizziness of freedom'—a freedom to choose, to have options, we must first have in place a capacity to tolerate overwhelming degrees of anxiety that are powerfully present in those earliest moments of life. As we have seen, this capacity is not the one that we can acquire alone. In such moments it is necessary that we are in the presence of a willing and curious mind that can offer reverie to our most primitive fear and anxieties often originating from within.

As we have seen, Klein [9] speaks of the importance for development of being able to reach the depression position. With the advent of this phase come the experience of depressive anxiety and an inclination for reparation, which psychoanalysts argue that is essential for the development of our creative capacities. When Kierkegaard wrote of those having learned to be anxious in the 'right way', we might think he is referring to those who can tolerate and be able to modify states of high anxiety without recourse to expulsion through action and doing, without prematurely reaching out for 'fact or reason'.

This chapter has explored those seminal, early experiences between mother and infant that are elemental to the binding and transforming of anxiety and thus creating anxiety of the 'right kind'. The right kind of anxiety is that which has been worked upon, made optimum in its intensity, yet whose presence I have argued is paramount for processes of sublimation, symbolisation and expression (through language, writing, art or music) to take place. We have explored what the consequences for development are for those whose anxiety has been left unbound—anxiety which subsequently overwhelms and stultifies development. For those who have not had conferred on them the early experience of a reposeful mind of a parent-figure, we should not feel too despairing as there are interventions that can make a difference. Anxiety states can be optimised; development can become unstuck when there is access to a mind that can contain, tolerate and transform the intolerable and the unthinkable.

With the current prevalence of patients presenting with anxiety to mental health clinics throughout Europe, we might draw upon Bion's idea of container/contained to understand, or indeed question, Western societies communal approach to the containment of anxiety as it has been explored in this chapter. Bion was keen to emphasise that it is not simply the mother or parent-figure that provides such a process of containment—this is also facilitated by the family, the school, the place of work and indeed the society as a whole. With current epidemic levels of anxiety in our society, we must wonder if institutions, organisations, government and our society as a whole provide enough containing function to its citizens in order to help ameliorate such primitive anxieties as have been explored in this chapter. Or perhaps worse still—do we increasingly live in societies whose values only serve to increase anxiety and arousal levels through its noncontainment?

Author details

Peter Slater
Tavistock Clinic, London, UK

*Address all correspondence to: peter.slater7@btopenworld.com

References

[1] Kierkegaard S. The Concept of Anxiety. New York: Liverlight; 2014. p. 188

[2] Mawson C. Psychoanalysis and Anxiety: From Knowing to Being. Abingdon: Routledge; 2019. pp. 3-16

[3] Bion WR. All My Sins Remembered: Another Part of a Life and the Other Side of Genius. London: Karnac; 1985. p. 173

[4] Freud S. Formulations on the Two Principles of Mental Functioning. The Standard Edition of the Complete Psychological Works of Sigmund Freud. Vol. 12. London: Hogarth Press; 1911

[5] Klein M. Notes on some schizoid mechanisms. In: Envy and Gratitude and Other Works. London: Hogarth Press; 1975. pp. 1-25

[6] Klein M. On the theory of anxiety and guilt. In: Envy and Gratitude and Other Works. London: Hogarth Press; 1975. p. 29

[7] Riviere J. The unconscious phantasy of an inner world reflected in examples from English literature. The International Journal of Psycho-Analysis. 1952;**33**:160-172

[8] Klein M. The importance of symbol formation in the development of the ego. In: Love Guilt and Reparation and Other Works. London: Hogarth Press; 1975. pp. 219-233

[9] Klein M. The mourning and it's relation to manic-depressive states. In: Love Guilt and Reparation and Other Works. London: Hogarth Press; 1975. pp. 344-370

[10] Halton W. Some unconscious aspects of organisational life: Contributions from psychoanalysis. In: Obholzer A, Roberts VZ, editors. Unconscious at Work. London: Routledge; 1994. pp. 11-19

[11] Yerkes RM, Dodson JD. The relation of strength of stimulus to rapidity of habit-formation. Journal of Comparative Neurology and Psychology. 1908;**18**:459-482. DOI: 10.1002/cne.920180503

[12] Bion WR. Learning from Experience. London: Karnac Books; 1962. p. 41

[13] Bion WR. The psychoanalytic study of thinking. The International Journal of Psychoanalysis. 1962;**43**:306-310

[14] Keats J. Letter to George and Thomas Keats. In: Rollins HE, editor. The Letters of John Keats. Vol. 1. Boston, MA: Harvard University Press; 1958

Chapter 10

Association between Bipolar Affective Disorder and Periodontal Diseases

Fernando Oliveira Costa, Fabiano Cunha and Rafael Lima

Abstract

Periodontitis, an inflammatory disease of periodontal tissues, is characterized by the progressive loss of support tissue and the insertion of teeth. It derives from the infection and interaction of specific bacterial species with host response components in susceptible individuals. A growing number of observational and epidemiological studies have been published, in the last decades, pointing to a possible association between stress, anxiety, and depression with the development and progression of periodontal diseases. One of the possible mechanisms of influence of stress and of the psychosocial factors, in the periodontal conditions, is the modification of the individual's behavior. The studies that assessed the association between stress, depression, and periodontal disease are numerous in different types of design, yet their data are still conflicting. Another recurrent serious condition of mental health, frequently associated with high rates of morbidity and mortality, is the bipolar affective disorder (BPAD). Although little investigated and with conflicting data, BPAD is a behavioral factor associated to the periodontal disease. In addition, little is known about its interference with the microbial and immunological response to periodontitis. The aim of this chapter is to describe the main scientific evidence of the association between BPAD and periodontitis.

Keywords: periodontal disease, bipolar affective disorder, tooth loss

1. Introduction

Periodontitis, an inflammatory disease of periodontal tissues, is characterized by the progressive loss of support tissue and the insertion of teeth (**Figure 1**). It derives from the infection and interaction of specific bacterial species with host response components in susceptible individuals [1].

A growing number of observational and epidemiological studies have been published, in the last decades, pointing to a possible association between stress, anxiety, and depression with the development and progression of periodontal diseases [2–4].

One of the possible mechanisms of influence of stress and of the psychosocial factors, in the periodontal conditions, is the modification of the individual's behavior. Individuals with high levels of stress tend to assume behaviors and habits which increase the risk of developing of several diseases, including periodontitis.

Individuals, in these conditions, tend to be more negligent in their oral hygiene, perhaps start or intensify the habit of smoking, or modify their nutritional habits with deleterious reflexes in the functions of their immunological system. Such conditions would entail predisposition to a greater gravity of periodontitis [3, 4].

It is known that the primary etiology of periodontitis is related to the accumulation of bacterial biofilm, given that certain bacterial species and their virulence factors are directly related to susceptibility, installation, and progression of the periodontitis [5]. Socransky et al. [6] analyzed the grouping of bacterial species in subgingival biofilms and determined six "bacterial complexes" grouped and classified by color (**Figure 2**). From these, the pathogens of red complex *Porphyromonas*

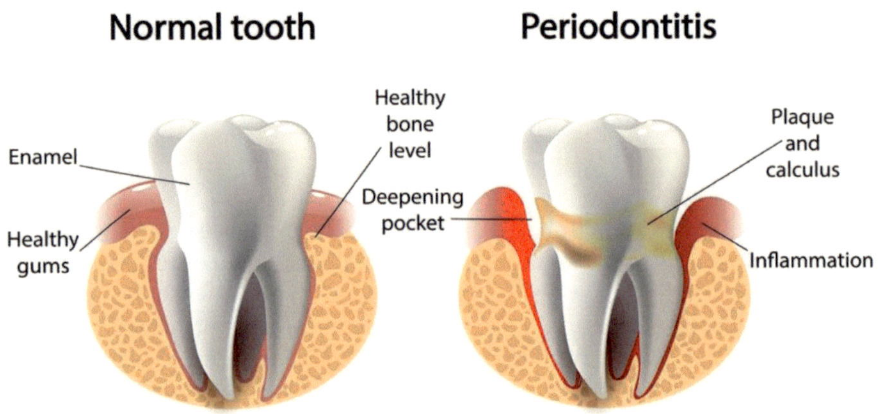

Figure 1.
Normal tooth x periodontitis.

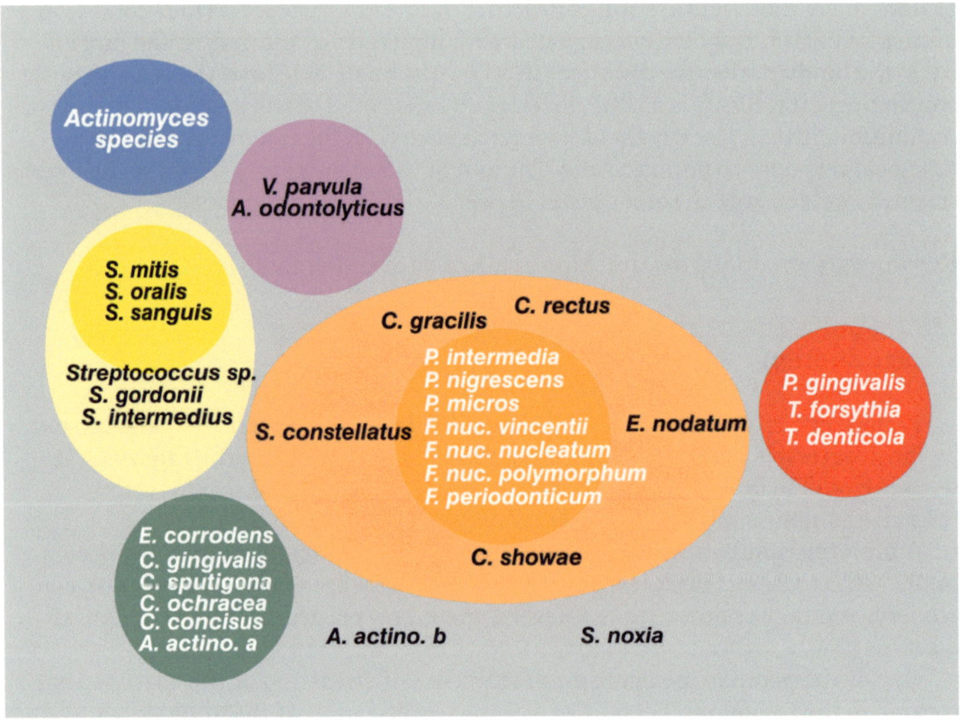

Figure 2.
Subgingival microbial complexes.

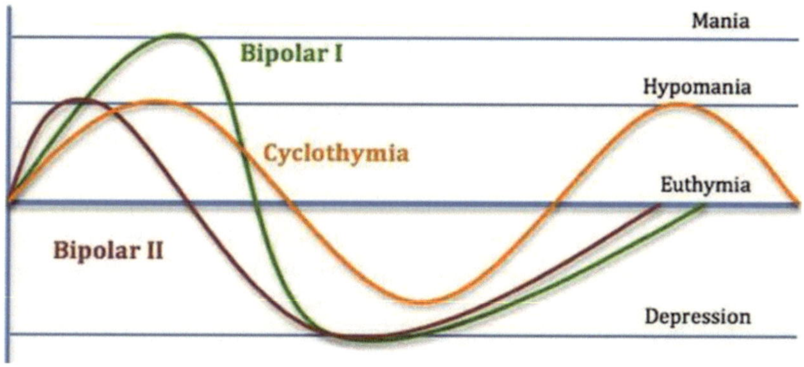

Figure 3.
States of humor in bipolar disorders.

gingivalis, *Treponema denticola*, and *Tannerella forsythia* have had an important association with periodontitis and *Aggregatibacter actinomycetemcomitans* which have been presented with a direct association with the type, gravity, and progression of periodontitis [5, 7]. Additionally, the bacteria of the red complex were also related to bigger depth of probing and bleeding on probing [6].

The studies that assessed the association between stress, depression, and periodontal disease are numerous in different types of design, yet their data are still conflicting [2–4, 8–17]. Another recurrent serious condition of mental health, frequently associated with high rates of morbidity and mortality, is the bipolar affective disorder (BPAD). The state of balance of mood, in the BPAD, is named euthymia. The term "thymia" comes from the ancient conception that the thymus, a gland located in the chest, would be responsible for the mood. Following this nomenclature, it is said that the mood (thymia), in a person with BPAD, suffers oscillations throughout the time. The normality is called euthymia, but when the mood is abnormally low, it is called depression, and when it is abnormally high, it is called mania. When the oscillations of mood are very marked with alternation of cycles, and go from great happiness to profound sadness, it is called cyclothymia. The alternation phases of depression with phases of mania characterize the BPAD, even though higher predominance and chronicity on stages of depression are observed [18, 19] (**Figure 3**).

Although little investigated and with conflicting data, bipolar affective disorder is a behavioral factor associated to the periodontal disease. In addition, little is known about its interference with the microbial and immunological response to periodontitis.

The aim of this chapter is to describe the main scientific evidence of the association between bipolar affective disorder and periodontitis.

2. Psychosocial factors and periodontal disease

The relationship between psychiatric disorders, negative emotional states, stress, and periodontal disease has been proposed since the 1950s. One of the pioneering studies of armed forces recruits has shown that the psychological stress resulting from such recruitment has increased the prevalence of necrotizing ulcerative gingivitis (GUN) in these individuals [20].

Some authors found that the severity of periodontal disease was greater in psychiatric subjects than in controls and that this severity was even greater among individuals with higher anxiety levels [21].

With the improvement of the laboratory techniques, some studies sought to measure corticoid levels in the urine, relating them to GUN episodes. Shannon et al. [22] found, in individuals with GUN, higher levels of corticosteroids than in controls, but this difference was not statistically significant. Maupin and Bell [23] found significantly elevated levels of corticosteroids during the course of GUN than after disease. Although these works provided a scientific basis for the relationships between emotional states and periodontal diseases, understanding of the time was limited. It was not yet known that some factors could interfere with emotional states, such as sports and social support, and periodontal disease, such as smoking and diabetes. Even the objective instruments of stress measurement were beginning to be elaborated. In the area of dentistry, it took some time for research to re-examine the association of psychosocial factors with periodontal disease.

One of the first studies that evaluated the possible association of stressful events with gingivitis and periodontitis was developed by Green et al. [24]. This study evaluated war veterans between the ages of 23 and 74 who sought emergency or routine care at the Brooklyn Veterans Dental Clinic. These individuals had somatic symptoms, probably from stressful situations. Self-report questionnaires were used to quantify the number of stressful events (Life Experiences Survey) and the number of somatic symptoms (Brief Symptom Inventory), with the objective of perceiving organic dysfunctions, including cardiovascular, respiratory, and intestinal symptoms, among others. According to the authors, gingivitis and periodontitis were found in more severe levels in individuals with high stress scores. It was concluded that there may be a correlation of the severity of gingivitis and periodontitis with the number of negative life events.

Freeman and Goss [25] retrospectively investigated some aspects of occupational stress on periodontal health using the Occupational Stress Indicator [26]. This instrument consists of a series of questions that measure the following aspects: personality type, job satisfaction, mental illness, and perception of physical illnesses. Among the advantages of this instrument is the access to the results of acute and chronic stress parameters, associated with life at work, as well as the possibility of relating these parameters to physical and mental well-being. After applying a regression model, there was a significant association of the increase in depth on probing with high levels of occupational stress (perception of physical stress symptoms) as well as the maintenance of a better periodontal health status in those who had positive behaviors and general health.

One study examined the association between occupational stress and the progression of periodontitis in employed adults. Individuals, regular dental followers (n = 23), were examined in two occasions (baseline and 5 years after the initial examination). Clinical measurements of periodontal condition, including clinical attachment loss, were made at four proximal sites on all teeth. A questionnaire, the Occupational Stress Indicator, was used to evaluate the stress retrospectively. The mean change in clinical attachment loss was 3 mm between the assessment periods. Multiple regression analysis was used to explore the relationship between clinical attachment loss, occupational stress measures, and sociodemographic data. In the final regression model, an increase in clinical attachment loss was significantly associated with increased age, lower socioeconomic status, and job dissatisfaction. According to the authors, the results suggest that occupational stress may have a relationship with the progression of periodontitis [27].

Monteiro da Silva et al. [28] verified the influence of psychosocial variables on individuals with periodontitis with rapid progression, adult periodontitis, and individuals without periodontal destruction. Psychological measures consisted of a life events scale, a University of California, Los Angeles (UCLA) solitude scale, and a somatization scale. The results showed an association between the symptoms of depression and the level of loneliness with periodontitis with rapid progression. Despite this, there was no association with adult periodontitis, currently classified as chronic periodontitis.

Araujo et al. [29] carried out a systematic review and meta-analysis, aiming to assess the scientific evidence on the association between depression and periodontitis. After selecting the studies, 15 were included in the systematic review (8 cross-sectional, 6 case–controls, and 1 cohort study). Six studies reported that depression was associated with periodontitis, whereas nine studies did not. The majority of studies had low risk of bias by methodological quality assessment. Meta-analysis of seven cross-sectional studies showed no significant association between depression and periodontitis (OR = 1.03, 95%, CI = 0.75–1.41). Findings from the present systematic review showed great heterogeneity among the studies, and the summary effect measure of the meta-analysis cannot affirm an association between depression and periodontitis. According to the authors, future studies with different designs in distinct populations should be conducted to investigate this association.

3. Bipolar affective disorder and periodontal disease

BPAD affects 1% of the population of the United States. These people suffer from episodes of extreme euphoria, followed by long periods of depression. A study was carried out in 40 individuals with BPAD diagnosis. They were submitted to oral health assessments regarding the presence of cavities, plaque index, and number of missing teeth. Poor oral hygiene, supra- and subgingival calculus accumulation, extensive dental caries, and numerous missing teeth were commonly identified in these individuals [30].

Chronic mental illness, and its treatment, carries inherent risks for important oral diseases. One of these groups is composed of individuals with BPAD. Through a combination of psychotherapy, pharmacotherapy, life adjustment, and multidisciplinary counseling, these individuals are better able to understand and deal with the underlying mood changes that characterize the condition and in turn interact more positively and progressively within society as a whole. Individuals with BPAD may exhibit various oral changes. These include the formation of root caries and periodontal disease [30, 31]. These diseases are related to the frequent neglect of oral hygiene care and the use of medications, especially lithium, which is related to side effects such as xerostomia. During the manic phase of BPAD (hyperactivity, euphoria), individuals tend to exacerbate oral hygiene care, predisposing to the appearance of abrasive lesions on the teeth, as well as gingival recessions. The knowledge by the dentists of this mental health disorder is essential for the establishment of correct management in the prevention and treatment of oral alterations commonly found in this group of individuals [31, 32].

A prevalence study of systemic diseases was carried out in individuals from a dental school, where 508 individuals were selected and answered a questionnaire for psychiatric evaluation. One hundred thirty-six individuals (26.77%) reported having at least one mental disorder. Of all the systemic disorders, depression was in second place in frequency, behind only hypertension. Drug abuse, anxiety, anorexia, bulimia, insomnia, bipolar affective disorder, and posttraumatic stress were also well reported. It was concluded that there is a need for training for dentistry students, with the aim of recognizing signs of psychiatric disorders in their individuals. The curriculum of dentistry should include this knowledge [33].

Caries and periodontal disease are common findings in individuals with BPAD. These changes have a negative impact on the quality of life and, often, on the response to psychiatric treatment [34].

The prevalence of psychiatric disorders was determined in adults undergoing dental treatment. Four hundred twenty-two subjects were selected in a college of dentistry through the evaluation of histories of psychiatric conditions. The most common disorder was depression. Other disorders included anxiety, bipolar affective disorder, attention deficit disorder, and schizophrenia. More than one disorder was found in 50% of men and 37% of women, and the most common condition was depression, along with anxiety. Seventy-seven percent of the women and 69% of the men, under these conditions, were under active treatment. The most common medications prescribed were serotonin reuptake inhibitors, benzodiazepines, lithium, and tricyclic antidepressants. Twenty individuals reported using more than one medication. It was concluded that a significant number of individuals, under dental care, present psychiatric disorders. These disorders can affect the response of individuals to dental treatment, requiring modifications in these treatments. The side effects of the drugs commonly used by these individuals may make it difficult to control oral hygiene of the same [35].

The prevalence of periodontal disease is generally higher because of poor oral hygiene and drug-induced xerostomia used by individuals with BPAD. Preventive dentistry education, saliva substitutes, and anti-caries agents are indicated. To avoid adverse drug interactions with commonly prescribed psychiatric medications, special precautions should be taken when administering certain antibiotics, analgesics, and sedatives [36].

Cunha et al. [37] evaluated the periodontal clinical condition and epidemiological and microbiological aspects of individuals with bipolar affective disorder. A convenience sample consisting of 156 participants with a diagnosis of BPAD, of both genders, was selected and submitted to complete and microbiological periodontal examination. Bleeding on probing (BOP), probing depth (PD), and clinical insertion level (CAL) on all teeth present were collected. Quantification of bacterial total charge and *Aggregatibacter actinomycetemcomitans*, *Treponema denticola*, *Tannerella forsythia*, and *Porphyromonas gingivalis* was performed by means of qPCR. The results showed a high prevalence of periodontitis (56.8%),

Study group	Phase of BPAD			P
	Mania	Euthymia	Depression	
Periodontitis				
No (n = 64; 43.2%)	20 (71.4%)	42 (46.2%)	2 (5.4%)	<0.001[A]
Yes (n = 92; 56.8%)	8 (28.6%)	49 (53.8%)	35 (94.6%)	
Total 156	28	91	37	
Severity				
Moderate (n = 83; 90.2%)	7 (87.5%)	43 (87.8%)	33 (94.3%)	0.483[B]
Advanced (n = 9; 9.8%)	1 (12.5%)	6 (12.2%)	2 (5.7%)	
Total 156	8	49	35	
Extension				
Localized (n = 75; 81.5%)	8 (100.0%)	40 (91.6%)	27 (77.1%)	0.439[B]
Generalized (n = 17; 18.5%)	0 (0.0%)	9 (18.4%)	8 (22.9%)	
Total 156	8	49	35	

[A]*Cunha et al. Chi-square test.*
[B]*Cunha et al. Fisher's exact test.*

Table 1.
Diagnosis, extent, and severity of periodontitis, related to phase of the BPAD.

the majority of which were chronic (90.2%) and localized (81.5%). The depressive phase in individuals with BPAD was strongly associated with the occurrence of periodontitis ($p < 0.001$). The specific bacterial count of *Treponema denticola*, *Tannerella forsythia*, *Porphyromonas gingivalis*, and red complex was significantly higher in individuals with BPAD and periodontitis, compared to the group with BPAD and without periodontitis. The percentage of sites with BOP and PD $\geq$ 4 mm showed a significant and positive correlation with the count of *Porphyromonas gingivalis*, *Treponema denticola*, and *Tannerella forsythia*. The final multivariate logistic regression model revealed that the probability of an individual with BPAD having periodontitis was higher in the depression phase (OR = 28.94, 95%, CI = 4.44–177.27, $p < 0.001$) than in the mania phase (OR = 1.91, 95%, CI = 1.0–1.99, $p < 0.001$) and the presence of a higher total bacterial load (OR = 1.91). It was concluded that individuals with BPAD presented a high prevalence of periodontitis and a higher frequency of periodontal diseases studied, confirming the importance of the need for prevention, diagnosis, and treatment of periodontitis, suggesting that this is a comorbidity associated with BPAD (**Table 1**).

4. Final considerations

BPAD is a complex psychiatric disorder characterized by the alternance of phases of mania and depression. It is frequently associated with metabolic and endocrinology disorders, and thus it must not be considered a disease that "only" affects the mood [31–34]. As the BPAD and the periodontitis are chronic diseases, presenting a big impact on the health and quality of life of individuals [1, 4, 7, 8], the present study aimed at evaluating the main aspects of association between these two important diseases.

This factor has great relevance because several studies [9, 11, 13, 36–38] that evaluated the association between psychosocial factors and periodontitis utilized retrospective data obtained from medical records or individuals without medical clinic experience to obtain the diagnosis of psychiatric disorders. In these studies [11, 13, 38], many times, the researcher himself (dental surgeon) applied the test/questionnaire of depressive-maniac symptoms in the selected sample, through a quantitative analysis (scores), and the diagnosis of mental health was determined. This strategy to sampling may affect, sensibly, the correct diagnosis of mental health of individuals and, consequently, the analysis, results, and conclusions of the research.

The literature presents few studies that evaluated dental health condition and BPAD [20–22, 24]. Cavity and periodontal disease were commonly found in groups of individuals with BPAD that had gone through dental evaluations [20–24]. Poor oral hygiene related to the behavioral profile of individuals with BPAD and the xerostomia induced by medicines with lithium are mentioned as possible factors associated with a worse condition of oral and periodontal health in this group of individuals [20, 21].

To date, only a scientific study [29] has compared the frequency of periodontopathogens in individuals with and without bipolar affective disorder with periodontitis. The results demonstrated an influence of the periodontitis in the count of the total bacterial load. Individuals with BPAD and periodontitis showed an expressive and significantly higher count than individuals with BPD and without periodontitis, both in relation to the presence of *P. gingivalis*, *T. denticola*, *T. forsythia*, *A. actinomycetemcomitans*, and red complex but also in the total bacterial load. Data from different studies corroborate our findings [5–7].

Individuals in the depression phase were the ones who presented the highest percentage of periodontitis (94,6%) in comparison with individuals in the mania phase (28,6%), Additionally, in the global sample, a bigger bacterial total load, higher levels of *T. denticola*, and red complex in individuals in the depression phase in comparison with the individuals in the euthymia and mania phases were observed. In the multivariate model, the evaluation of the reason of chance revealed that the individuals in the depression phase had 28,04 more chance of having periodontitis than an individual in the mania phase [29].

Besides that, we can hypothetically assume that during depressive episodes, individuals with BPAD may present a decline in the level of oral hygiene. On the other hand, during the periods of mania, there can be an exacerbation in oral hygiene care. According to Friedlander and Birch [21], the mania phase is associated with an increase in the incidence and gravity of cervical abrasive lesions and gingival lacerations. According to Croucher et al. [38], poor oral hygiene, the accumulation of supra- and subgingival calculus, extensive dental cavities, and numerous lost teeth were commonly identified in the depressed individuals. In this line of thinking, individuals with BPAD with exacerbation of the mania phase could increase oral hygiene care in comparison with individuals in the exacerbated depression phase and thus impact positively the periodontal clinical parameters. However, one study [29] with a transversal design cannot confirm these findings because our results refer to the moment of the exam and must not be extrapolated to long-term conditions. In this sense, additional studies with representative samples and longitudinal monitoring are necessary to confirm if the different phases of the mental state present in the BPAD could influence the present and progression of the periodontitis.

In this sense, we indicate that patients with BPAD have an unsatisfactory oral condition, characterized mainly by the presence of periodontal diseases and tooth loss. These poor oral conditions negatively impact the quality of life of these patients. Dentists should alert psychiatrists, nurses, social workers, and caregivers to the need for good oral hygiene, including proper brushing, flossing, and use of coadjuvants such as oral irrigators and interdental brushes. Thus, it is necessary to carry out actions in oral health, preventive and curative, for this vulnerable population. In addition, it is important to regularly visit the dentist and establish a good oral health program aimed at improving the quality of life of the population suffering from mental and behavioral disorders.

Author details

Fernando Oliveira Costa*, Fabiano Cunha and Rafael Lima
Federal University of Minas Gerais, Belo Horizonte, Brazil

*Address all correspondence to: focperio@uol.com.br

References

[1] American Academy of Periodontology. Task force report on the update to the 1999 classification of periodontal diseases and conditions. Journal of Periodontology. 2015;**86**:1-5

[2] Moss ME, Beck JD, Kaplan BH. Exploratory case control analysis of psychosocial factors and adult periodontitis. Journal of Clinical Periodontology. 1996;**67**:1060-1069

[3] Genco RJ, Ho AW, Grossi SG, Dunford RG, Tedesco LA. Relationship of stress, distress, and inadequate coping behaviors to periodontal disease. Journal of Periodontology. 1999;**70**:711-723

[4] Hugoson A, Ljungquist B, Breivik T. The relationship of some negative life events and psychological factors to periodontal disease in an adult: Swedish population 50 to 80 years of age. Journal of Clinical Periodontology. 2002;**29**:247-253

[5] Haffajee AD, Bogren A, Hasturk H, Feres M, Lopez NJ, Socransky SS. Subgingival microbiota of chronic periodontitis subjects from different geographic locations. Journal of Clinical Periodontology. 2004;**31**:996-1002

[6] Socransky SS, Haffajee AD, Cugini MA, Smith C, Kent RL. Microbial complexes in subgingival plaque. Journal of Clinical Periodontology. 1998;**25**:134-144

[7] Cortelli JR, Cortelli SC, Jordan S, Haraszthy VI, Zambon JJ. Prevalence of periodontal pathogens in Brazilians with aggressive or chronic periodontitis. Journal of Clinical Periodontology. 2005;**32**(8):860-866

[8] Pearson GR, Persson RE, MacEntee CI, Wyatt CC, Hollender LG, Kiyak HA. Periodontitis and perceived risk for periodontitis in elders with evidence of depression. Journal of Clinical Periodontology. 2003;**30**:691-696

[9] Saletu A, Pirker H, Saletu F, Linzmayer L, Anderer P, Matejka M. Controlled clinical and psychometric studies on the relation between periodontitis and depressive mood. Journal of Clinical Periodontology. 2005;**32**:1219-1225

[10] Castro GD, Opperman RV, Haas AN, Winter R, Alchieri JC. Association between psychosocial factors and periodontitis: A case control study. Journal of Clinical Periodontology. 2006;**33**:109-114

[11] Ng SKS, Leung WK. A community study on the relationship between stress, coping, affective dispositions and periodontal attachment loss. Community Dentistry and Oral Epidemiology. 2006;**34**:252-266

[12] Johannsen A, Rydmark I, Soder B, Asberg M. Gingival inflammation, increased periodontal pocket depth and elevated interleukin-6 in gingival crevicular fluid of depressed women on long-term sick leave. Journal of Periodontal Research. 2007;**42**:546-552

[13] Rosania AE, Low KG, Mc Cormick CM, Rosania DA. Stress, depression, cortisol and periodontal disease. Journal of Periodontology. 2009;**80**:260-266

[14] Abahneh KT, All Shaar MB, Taani DQ. Depressive symptoms in relation periodontal health in a Jordanian sample. International Journal of Dental Hygiene. 2010;**8**:16-21

[15] Solis AC, Marques AH, Pannuti CM, Lotufo RF, Lotufo-Neto F. Evaluation of periodontitis in hospital outpatients

with major depressive disorder. Journal of Periodontal Research. 2014;**49**:77-84

[16] Warren KR, Postolache TT, Groer ME, Pinjari O, Kelly DL, Reynolds MA. Role of chronic stress and depression in periodontal diseases. Periodontology 2000. 2014;**2000, 64**:127-138

[17] Araujo MM, Martins CC, Costa LC, Cota LO, Faria RL, Cunha FA, et al. Association between depression and periodontitis: A systematic review and meta-analysis. Journal of Clinical Periodontology. 2016;**43**:216-228

[18] Perry W, McIlwain M, Kloezeman K, Henry BL, Minassian A. Diagnosis and characterization of mania: Quantifying increased energy and activity in the human behavioral pattern monitor. Psychiatry Research. 2016;**23**:278-283

[19] Samalin L, Reinares M, de Chazeron I. Course of residual symptoms according to the duration of euthymia in remitted bipolar patients. Acta Psychiatrica Scandinavica. 2016;**134**:57-64. DOI: 10.1111/acps.12568

[20] Johnson BD, Engel D. Acute necrotizing ulcerative gingivitis. A review of diagnosis, etiology and treatment. Journal of Periodontology. 1986;**57**:141-150

[21] Friedlander AH, Birch NJ. Dental conditions in patients with bipolar disorder on long-term lithium maintenance therapy. Special Care in Dentistry. 2009;**10**:148-151

[22] Shannon IL, Kilgore WG, O'Leary TJ. Stress as a predisposing factor in necrotizing ulcerative gingivitis. Journal of Periodontology. 1969;**40**:240-242

[23] Maupin CC, Bell WB. The relationship of 17-hydroxycorticosteroid to acute necrotizing ulcerative gingivitis. Journal of Periodontology. 1975;**46**:721-722

[24] Green LW, Tryon WW, Marks B, Huryn J. Periodontal disease as a function of life events stress. Journal of Human Stress. 1986;**12**:32-36

[25] Freeman R, Goss S. Stress measures as predictors of periodontal disease-a preliminary communication. Community Dental Oral Epidemiology. 1993;**21**:176-177

[26] Cooper CL, Baglioni AJ Jr. A structural model approach toward the development of a theory of the link between stress and mental health. Brazilian Journal Medical Psychology. 1988;**61**:87-102

[27] Linden GJ, Mullally BH, Freeman R. Stress and the progression of periodontal disease. Journal of Clinical Periodontology. 1996;**23**:675-680

[28] Monteiro da Silva AM, Oakley DA, Newman HN, Noh FS, Loyd HM. Psychosocial factors and adult onset rapidly progressive periodontitis. Journal of Clinical Periodontology. 1996;**23**:789-794

[29] Araújo MM, Martins CC, Costa LC, Cota LO, Faria RL, Cunha FA, et al. Association between depression and periodontitis: A systematic review and meta-analysis. Journal of Clinical Periodontology. 2016;**43**(3):216-228

[30] Pavlova B, Perlis RH, Mantere O, Sellgren CM, Isometsä E, Mitchell PB, et al. Prevalence of current anxiety disorders in people with bipolar disorder during euthymia: A meta-analysis. Psychological Medicine. 2017;**47**(6):1107-1115

[31] Giglio JA, Laskin DM. Prevalence of psychiatric disorders in a group of

adult patients seeking general dental care. Quintessence International. 2010;**41**:433-437

[32] Clark DB. Dental care for the patient with bipolar disorder. Journal of the Canadian Dental Association. 2003;**69**:20-24

[33] Woods CD. Self-reported mental illness in a dental school clinic population. Journal of Dental Education. 2003;**67**:500-504

[34] Friedlander AH, Birch NJ. Dental conditions in patients with bipolar disorder on long-term lithium maintenance therapy. Special Care in Dentistry. 2009;**10**:148-151

[35] Giglio JA, Laskin DM. Prevalence of psychiatric disorders in a group of adult patients seeking general dental care. Quintessence International. 2010;**41**:433-437

[36] Beltrán-Aguilar ED, Eke PI, Thornton-Evans G, Petersen PE. Recording and surveillance systems for periodontal diseases. Periodontology 2000. 2012;**60**:40-53

[37] Cunha FA, Cota LOM, Cortelli SC, Miranda TB, Neves FS, Cortelli JR, et al. Periodontal condition and levels of bacteria associated with periodontitis in individuals with bipolar affective disorders: A case-control study. Journal of Periodontal Research. 2019;**54**(1):63-72

[38] Croucher R, Marcenes WS, Torres MC, Hughes WS. The relationship between life-events and periodontitis. A case control study. Journal of Clinical Periodontology. 1997;**24**:39-47